Against Doctor's Orders

Against Doctor's Orders

Ali Weinberg Barton

WiDō Publishing
Salt Lake City • Houston

WiDō Publishing
Salt Lake City, Utah
widopublishing.com

Cover design by Steven Novak
Photography by Kevan Gale and by Tracy Rodriguez Photography
Book design by Marny K. Parkin

ISBN: 978-1-937178-83-3
Library of Congress Control Number available upon request

Printed in the United States of America

This book is dedicated to Ethan.
You are my light and love, and you bring me endless joy.
I would do it all over again in a heartbeat.

And to my donor,
for blessing me with a second chance at life.

In honor of Grandma Sylvia and Grandma Estelle

Chapter One

The Fertility Consult

I SAT IN MY JOHNNIE IN THE REPRODUCTIVE ENDO-crinologist's office, waiting for the doctor to come in after my exam. My hands shook with anxiety, my mind racing with hope and doubt. I prayed that she would approve me for the procedure. My eyes gazed over the room, as I did not want to move from my spot on the exam table to reach for a magazine. I looked at the walls covered in posters and pamphlets about menstrual cycles, in vitro fertilization, and infertility. I felt my eyes welling up with tears and resentment that I needed to go down this path.

My husband Andrew sat in a chair across from me, stiff with discomfort. I knew we would need fertility treatments, since my cycle had been abnormal ever since I had gotten sick with autoimmune problems a few years earlier. I hated dragging Andrew to this office.

"Well, Allison. I think you could be a good candidate for the IVF based on the exam. I get nervous about your past heart issue, and I am going to need to talk to your cardiologist prior to beginning an IVF cycle with you. I also want you to have a consult with maternal fetal medicine to clear you for this."

I nodded my head and reached for my husband Andrew's hand. The heart issue. It had come back to haunt me again, and I was prepared with an answer.

"I totally understand. We already had a meeting last month with my cardiologist to discuss the safety of getting pregnant, and he gave us the okay. He said he would be happy to talk to you about it."

"I also think it can't hurt to gain a few pounds and relax on the exercise," the doctor continued. "Some women with hypothalamic amenorrhea just need a higher body fat percentage and then they have an easier time getting pregnant."

I nodded. "I know, I have read that. I promise you I am eating more and working out less."

After reading about hypothalamic amenorhhea two months prior, I had committed to moving less and increasing calories, but it caused me tremendous anxiety. I loved teaching fitness and yoga, and it was difficult for me to "be lazy," as I saw it, and not exercise every day. I felt comfortable and safe with my strict paleo diet and staunchly believed it had healed my autoimmune issues. I made a mental note to eat ice cream and more almond butter and avocados in the following weeks.

Chapter 2

The Sick Girl

ANDREW HAD BEEN WORRIED SINCE DAY ONE about having the baby discussion. Ever since I had developed heart issues back in 2010, he worried about my health and survival.

Andrew and I had only been dating for eight months when I started to notice odd and sometimes painful symptoms. I was working full time as a licensed mental health counselor for families and children, and had a part time job as a fitness instructor and yoga teacher, something I'd done for ten years. At twenty-eight, I was active and healthy, but I began to notice that simple movement was causing exhaustion.

My heart rate would skyrocket to 200 when I walked up a flight of stairs, and I would need to rest at the top. I felt breathless when teaching my classes and struggled to get up off the floor after playing with a child client. For weeks, I'd known something was wrong for weeks, but I hoped it was a virus that would go away on its own.

One weekend in July of 2010, I drove myself to the emergency room. Andrew was visiting his family in Vermont, and I was afraid I wouldn't make it through the night alive. When I lay down to sleep, the pain in my chest was too much to ignore. I thought I might have pulled a muscle in my chest while teaching a fitness class. Whatever it was, I knew I needed to get it checked out. I was concerned that I might even be having a heart attack.

The doctors confirmed I had something called pericarditis, which is inflammation around the heart. They said it was common for people to get a viral infection and develop this inflammation. They prescribed me a high dose anti-inflammatory and sent me home. My parents had rushed to the hospital, and Andrew had insisted on coming home. I was just happy to have a diagnosis and felt this was no big deal. I would be fine.

Weeks later, things were certainly not fine. My health had worsened, so the doctor thought that it was severe enough to warrant steroids. The next few months, I completed several rounds of steroid tapers, to only get sicker each time I came off the prednisone. Not only was I physically ill, I was an emotional mess. Prednisone made me a maniac. I could not sleep, I was hyper one minute, and sobbing the next.

I needed to take disability from work, and the doctors prescribed anti-anxiety medication to calm me down. For someone who exercised six days a week, I was instructed to stay put on the couch, and

I was devastated. I was also panicked about getting the infamous "moon face" and weight gain from steroids and decided to be stricter with monitoring my food intake.

One weekend in September, I went away with my family. I insisted I felt fine enough to go with everyone on a long bike ride. I felt like I'd die on that bike path. Not wanting to worry anyone, I kept it to myself and pushed through. Everyone completed the two hour-long bike ride with ease, while I struggled like someone who had never exercised a day in her life. That night, I looked in the mirror and didn't recognize myself. My body was puffy and swollen. When I stood for too long, my lower legs would swell up, and the pressure would be unbearable.

My stomach also bothered me on that trip, and I experienced flu-like symptoms. Later that week, after coming back home, Andrew took me to the ER in a panic. I felt as if I had an elephant sitting on my chest.

This time was different. The doctors seemed concerned, whispering in the hallways and watching my medical monitors. No one would tell me what was happening. Dozens of different doctors and nurses came into my room to do their evaluations as I sat terrified on my twin bed, my eyes darting around the room and sobbing to whoever would listen, "What's wrong with me?"

I cried to my family, who had rushed over when the doctors admitted me. "Why won't anyone tell me what is happening?"

Hours later, we found out I had developed a fibrous mass in my right ventricle; no one knew how or why it got there.

Over the course of the next week, I had biopsies, blood tests, CAT scans, MRIS, X RAYS, and other tests, with no conclusive answers coming back. Some doctors had hypothesized a rare disease called Hypereosinophilic Syndrome, but other specialists doubted this diagnosis to be true.

The case was presented at the Mayo Clinic, which further confirmed that my illness did not match this hypothesis. One doctor thought the mass was auto-immune related. He started me on a high dose of steroids and diuretics to help reduce the edema and swelling that was causing me such pain.

When things were under control, they sent me home on my medication, telling me the steroids would help to reduce the mass.

In the following weeks, I did more research on autoimmune conditions and read about how the different organs could be affected by autoimmune problems. My liver enzymes tested out of range too high, my stomach felt bloated and swollen (and had been this way since I was a child), my thyroid was not functioning well, I did not have a menstrual cycle, and now this heart problem was the worst of all of them. I feared I was going to die.

I decided to go gluten free. I did not know anything about gluten at this time, but the naturopathic medical articles that I read linked autoimmune

disease to intestinal permeability and gluten intol-
erance. Through the articles I learned that for some
people, gluten is difficult to digest; it enables the
tight junctions in the intestines to develop small
gaps. This allows food proteins to travel through
the gaps and into the bloodstream, where the body
could launch the autoimmune system to fight off the
foreign proteins that should not be in the system.

Within a week of going gluten free, I felt normal
again. My stomach was not bloated, and I had no
cramping after eating. I had been in pain for years,
and it was simply my normal. In the past, doctors
had diagnosed me with IBS and told me to eat more
fiber and to relax.

"I think I may have celiac," I told my immunologist one afternoon at a follow up appointment. He
drummed his fingers on his desk, and then stroked
his chin. I continued, "It makes total sense. All my
organs have been affected by my autoimmune disease. What if the heart was the last straw?"

I proceeded to tell him about my constant stomach, thyroid, liver, colon, and hyper pituitary adre-
nal axis dysregulation. I thought my heart problems
could be linked to having been undiagnosed celiac.

"And I feel much better being gluten free. Could
this be what caused the heart problem?"

He agreed this could potentially be true and set
me up for some more tests. "If you feel better being
gluten free, then keep doing it!" he encouraged me.

Over the course of the next few weeks I had an

endoscopy and colonoscopy, since blood tests had come back negative for celiac. Because I had chronic and dangerous low antibody levels that I'd later need IV infusions to increase, the antibody blood tests would not be accurate. I had been gluten free for several weeks, but I was not willing to do the gluten challenge—reintroduce large amounts of gluten to create further damage in the villi—for my results. Even with no gluten challenge, both sets indicated damage to my villi and confirmed the celiac diagnosis. The GI doctor had also ordered the genetic tests; all three tests came back indicating celiac disease.

I had felt wonderful and healthy on a gluten free diet. Since I had convinced myself that my autoimmune problems were caused by gluten, I would not change my diet.

Chapter 3

Celiac

I WAS READY TO PUT ALL THIS MEDICAL DRAMA behind me and move on with my life. The more research I did, the more it made sense that eating gluten all of these years had caused slow damage to many of my organs. I could not find research studies on the connection between heart problems and undiagnosed celiac disease, but I was on the mend and moving on.

I was still on disability from work. During my leave, I realized how my job working with challenging families drained me emotionally and physically. I was ready to make a career change.

"Why don't you complete the wellness coaching program?" Andrew asked me one afternoon, as we took the dog on a walk. He was referring to a health coaching program he'd completed in years prior.

I was getting back into doing yoga and would begin teaching yoga and fitness once I got clearance from my team. I thought this coaching would be a good fit with my career in mental health and fitness. I decided to do the course.

I missed movement and had a passion, if not addiction, to exercise. The last few months had me aching to move around again. The combination of prednisone, no appetite, and lack of physical activity caused me to look skinny and weak. My muscles had wasted away, and my clothes were huge on me. I couldn't wait to begin working out and teaching again. I struggled being at home on the couch every day, but my doctors did not want me returning to work. The course could help to keep my brain occupied.

Andrew owned his own company, Engin Coaching, where he did personal training and health coaching, and I felt envious of the work he did with his clients. I had often thought about starting my own private psychotherapy practice, but wanted to also find a way to incorporate my love for fitness, health, and nutrition into my career. This would be the way.

The more time I had, the more I stewed over how frustrated I felt with what had happened. I thought I took great care of myself. I ate healthy foods, exercised, did yoga and stress management, slept well, and socialized with good friends. All of the things "they" said to do. I felt a complete resentment towards my body for failing me and a sense of regret for not having my stomach problems checked out earlier. I was angry at my doctors for not giving me any answers about my illness. No one seemed to have a clue as to why I had gotten sick, but everyone seemed content with the fact that the mass in my heart was getting smaller. I wanted to learn more about coaching others with health issues, so that other people would not feel as lost and alone as I had felt. This course was the step I needed to take to keep myself busy and to feel productive.

As the months went by, I felt healthier, and returned to work with permission from the doctors. I went back part time, since I'd decided I wanted to start my own practice after I had passed the wellness coaching certification.

The practice started off slow and steady, but I felt ready to leave my job and go full time with my own business in the winter of 2011.

Chapter 4

Back to Life

LIFE WAS WONDERFUL. I HAD PERIODIC CHECK ups with my immunologist and cardiologist, and they seemed pleased that the heart seemed to be stable. Some days I would wake up feeling swollen and fatigued, and it would get worse as the day progressed. The cardiologist would give me diuretics, but it boggled my mind that I could wake up one day and be twelve to fifteen pounds heavier than the day before. For someone who had a lifelong struggle with body image and struggled with eating disorders in high school and college, this was pushing me over the edge. I felt puffy and insecure in my body.

My cardiologist thought there may be some damage from where the mass was. He added a diagnosis of tricuspid regurgitation, but he felt it was something that could be managed and regulated with careful monitoring and medications.

As a coping mechanism for dealing with the lack of control over my body, I became fixated on other things. One was getting married. I had known since my hospitalization in 2010 that I wanted to marry Andrew. I had felt like a sick and broken person then, and he assured me that he loved me regardless of my health status and would be happy with a life together even if I could not birth a child. I wanted to be a mother; I felt I was born to do so. At the time of the hospitalization, doctors doubted that I would be able to have children.

As the months passed, my cardiologist felt comfortable with my progress and health improvements. He told me when the time came, we could have a meeting to discuss pregnancy. I was thrilled.

Starting at the holidays of 2010, I had waited patiently for Andrew to propose. He was eleven years older, and I knew he would want to settle down soon. Every holiday and special occasion for the next two years left me sad and disappointed. Every time he reached into his pocket, I thought, "This is it!" We had talked about marriage, and we had moved in together after I got sick, but there was no follow through.

I promised myself I would not become one of "those girls," but here I was, first dropping subtle marriage hints and then turning into a mild nagger. I was starting to feel as if I was not good enough.

When he was first moving in, I asked him, "This is not going to turn into a 'why buy the cow if you can get the milk for free' situation, is it?"

He laughed and assured me it would not. Andrew had experienced some bad divorces with his parents and subsequent step-parents when he was a child, and I thought that perhaps he was too traumatized to want to marry me.

One afternoon, he got upset with me for pestering him. "Is it too much pressure for us to live together and not be married? Do I need to move out?"

I was shocked and startled by Andrew's statement, and in that moment I realized that I did not care about marriage. What I cared about was being with Andrew.

"Andrew, if marriage freaks you out that much, screw it! You are not moving out. I love you and we don't need to get married. All I want is you. We can have a life together without being married." I snuggled up on his lap and felt him breathe a sigh of relief. Part of me knew what I said was the truth, but still I was devastated. I knew I would not be satisfied without marriage.

Andrew acted strange for weeks after that day. He was quiet, pensive, and on his laptop in the office for hours at a time. I convinced myself that he was researching new places to live. I was in panic mode.

On New Year's Eve 2011, I woke up with a sore throat. I had planned on brunch with my girlfriends and decided to go despite not feeling great. I needed to vent to my girlfriends and wanted a little bit of space from Andrew.

We sat around the table in one of our favorite restaurants with salads the size of our heads, nachos, iced teas and champagne filling up the table. It was a sports bar, and I did not want to look like a desperate girl sobbing about her boyfriend.

"I know I said I was okay with not getting married, but I just don't think I am! I don't get why he doesn't want to marry me," I sobbed.

My girlfriends assured me that he would surprise me one day, along with all the other obligatory things girls need to say to one another in these moments. Within minutes, they had me giggling and forgetting about my sadness.

I went home after lunch feeling in a better emotional space but physically feverish and terrible. I came in the door and saw Andrew in the office. *Great,* I thought. *Probably looking for more apartments.*

"Hey, hon." He seemed distant and would not look up at me. I walked into the bedroom, peeled off my clothing, and threw on my ratty pajamas and robe.

Feeling sorry for myself, I lay down on the couch to enjoy some New Year's Day parades on TV. I said to Andrew, "Ugh, I feel like shit. I'm pretty sure I have a sinus infection."

"Hon, can I show you something?" He came over to me laptop in hand. I rolled my eyes. This was code for business talk. Andrew did a lot of behind the scenes work for our company and always wanted to share website stuff with me.

No! I thought. *Not in the mood.*

When he sat next to me, I noticed he was shaking. I had a moment of pure panic that he was about to break up with me.

"I know I have been acting weird the last few days, and I thought this would be here by now so I could do this tonight, but . . ." He turned the laptop around and showed me a picture of a stunning diamond ring.

"What?" I shrieked. He laughed.

"It was supposed to be delivered today, but it is not here, and I can't act normal without telling you what's going on. Will you marry me?"

I started laughing and crying at the same time. "I thought you were about to break up with me!"

We hugged and kissed, as I said "Yes! Of course!"

We made our calls to family and friends, and my girlfriends teased me for being so paranoid.

When the Fed Ex truck pulled up our street two days later, I was walking the dog. We lived at the top of a steep hill, and although I was not supposed to run, I sprinted up to chase the truck, ensuring I would not miss the delivery. I was out of breath, and my heart felt like it was going to explode. I assured myself that I was just out of shape, and nothing was wrong with my heart anymore.

Chapter 5

Getting Married

WITHIN THE NEXT TWO WEEKS, I FINISHED planning the entire wedding. Andrew's friends joked that I had already planned the event before we were engaged. That was my personality; I knew what I wanted and was persistent in getting my way. My parents saw this trait as annoying, stubborn, and difficult, but in my mind, it had worked wonders for me many times in my life. It would also prove to be to my advantage over the next few years.

We wanted a summer wedding, and I did not want to wait for another year and a half. Andrew was already forty, and I would be turning thirty. I wanted kids before it was too late.

We had a beautiful wedding on July 28, 2012, at the Hotel Marlowe in Cambridge, Massachusetts. I had surprised myself with how relaxed I was with the whole thing, even teaching a boot camp class the morning of the wedding. I was so excited to marry Andrew and start our lives together. I was eager to begin our family. Our friend Chris got ordained online, and we had a lighthearted and fun ceremony, despite the torrential downpour that happened minutes before our gorgeous, outdoor park wedding was scheduled to happen.

The months following our wedding felt like we were on fast forward. We stayed close to home for our honeymoon: Rhode Island and Maine, and planned a trip that winter to the Dominican. After returning home to our condo, we decided to start looking at new houses. We had talked about beginning a family, and I had set up an appointment with the fertility specialist after speaking with my PCP about our options for getting pregnant.

We fell in love with a beautiful old farmhouse outside of Boston, and decided it was our dream home. In September 2012, we made an offer, and it was accepted. At the same time, we had our appointment at the IVF clinic, and decided to begin our journey to getting pregnant in November.

Chapter 6

The IVF

AFTER THE MEETING WITH DR. ABNER, I WAS eager to start the process. We consulted again with my cardiologist, Dr. Levine. Andrew asked him, "Are you *sure* she will be okay getting pregnant?"

As the days passed, Andrew grew more concerned about my past heart issues and carrying a baby. Dr. Levine assured him I would be fine—perhaps get more edema than the average woman, but I would be fine. He told me I was "so healthy now".

We had our consult with the doctor in maternal fetal medicine, Dr. Economy. After she got the go ahead from Dr. Levine, we were ready to begin. I liked her personality from the moment I met her, and felt comforted knowing she would be keeping an eye on me during the pregnancy.

We planned on starting with the process of IUI (intra uterine insemination), and converting to IVF (in vitro fertilization) if I made too many eggs. Secretly, I was thrilled when this happened. I knew the chances of pregnancy were higher with the precision of IVF. The procedure and transfer both occurred in the week of our move. After doing research on the procedures, I knew it was not good to endure a large amount of physical or stress during IVF, but I have always been what my dad called a "right now-nick" and wanted to be pregnant as soon as I could.

I had such a good feeling about that first cycle. They went in and retrieved eleven eggs. I was devastated when I got the call telling me only two had fertilized. "If this doesn't work, next time we can do something called ICSI, where we directly inject the sperm into the egg to increase the chances of fertilization."

I prayed for those two eggs to implant and hoped it would result in twins. Two weeks after the transfer, amidst eager unpacking in our new house, I got the call from the clinic after getting my blood drawn that morning. "It's a positive!" I had peed on a stick the day before and seen a faint line. This was all the assurance I needed.

"We will need you to come back in two days for some more blood testing." I hung up the phone, screaming and crying. I called Andrew immediately, knowing he was with a client. He picked up, knowing I would either be sobbing or screaming. "Hello?" he asked nervously.

"It worked!" I screamed. "I'm pregnant!" We talked about my discussion with the clinic and promised a celebration dinner that night. I proceeded to call my parents, siblings, and best friends to tell them the great news. We were going to have a baby!

Two days later, while I was organizing the kitchen, the clinic called late afternoon, a few hours after I'd gone in for more blood testing.

"Allison, I am so sorry to tell you this. The HCG did not double. This is what we call a chemical pregnancy. Dr. Abner will call you later to discuss."

I sank down onto the floor, noticing some crumbs underneath the kitchen table. My dog Maddie came towards me to lick my hand. "I don't understand!" I sobbed into the phone. I had a client coming for a session in twenty minutes, and my world had just been turned upside down.

She proceeded to tell me this was very common with IVF, and since they test for pregnancy so early using this technique, there are more chemical pregnancies and miscarriages than an average woman would even know about. "Chromosomal abnormalities that make an embryo less able to survive tend to miscarry, and as far as a woman knows, she is having a period. It is a blessing and a curse to find out about a baby this early in a pregnancy."

I called Andrew, hysterical. I had no idea that the HCG needed to double and felt silly for not doing my research. Andrew came right home, and I cancelled my client session. The next few days I moped around, embarrassed for getting so excited so early on and sharing my news with so many people. I decided that the next cycle, I would just share with my family. I told Andrew I wanted to start it right away.

The next few months I walked around numb, with a dark cloud over my head. We did two more cycles pretty close together, and each time I did a cycle, we got fewer eggs. I felt like a complete and total failure.

"Maybe your body just needs a break, hon." Andrew gently suggested.

"No! I want to keep trying as many times as insurance will let us!"

The last cycle had been in March of 2013. I started the medication Lupron at the end of our delayed honeymoon in the Dominican Republic. By day three, I felt as if I had gained about twenty pounds. I was puffy, uncomfortable, and too embarrassed to put on a bathing suit. I would sit and look in the mirror before we would go out to dinner, knowing something was very wrong and trying to find baggy clothing to feel comfortable in.

I didn't want to ruin our trip, so I never complained about it, but Andrew knew I was not feeling well. I knew that I could have pretty exaggerated body dysmorphia at times, so I tried to let it go. I was sure I was having an allergic reaction to the medication, or I had accidentally eaten gluten. In retrospect, it was an indication of a problem with my heart. The fluid overload that I could accumulate overnight was astonishing. I called Dr. Levine's office from the Dominican, and he recommended taking extra diuretics. Dr. Abner's office told me to stop the medication, and we would take another approach.

When I got on the scale at home, I had gained twenty-one pounds, which vanished a week later with diuretics. Still, Dr. Levine ensured me I was fine, just a bad reaction to the medications. That IVF cycle failed, as I had predicted. Two out of three positive results, but no sticking embryos, and cycle three failing altogether.

Dr. Abner had us in her office one afternoon in the early spring of 2013. "Allison, I think you should consider using donor eggs. For some reason, these pregnancies won't stick. I think it may be an egg issue. Perhaps your autoimmune diseases impacted egg quality, or the functioning of your ovaries." Andrew grasped for my hand.

"But I am only thirty," I said. "Doesn't egg quality start to decline in your forties?" Tears started streaming down my face. At this point, I felt so much resentment for my medical issues. It seemed like all my friends were getting pregnant on their first try. Although my whole life had changed after getting sick in 2010, I'd stayed optimistic that it would not get in the way of being a mother.

"I think you may want to try another clinic then. I think we have done all we can here." I wiped my tears. Was I being fired by a reproductive endocrinologist? I wiped my tears and gathered my bag.

"Fine," I said, and walked out the door.

Andrew followed me and held me in a hug. "We can always adopt," he said, wiping my tears in the hallway. I knew this was an option, and I was not opposed to it, but was not ready to give up on IVF yet. The next day, I was on the phone with Dr. Ryley at Boston IVF, one of the city's best IVF clinics. He agreed to see us the following week.

I loved Dr. Ryley and felt confident that he could get me pregnant. He made me feel comfortable, and he had several ideas about approaching the cycle with different medication protocols.

"Allison, I will tell you this, though," he said, looking over his glasses at me, sitting with my hands clasped in a chair across from his desk, "I am not doing anything until I have that letter in hand from your cardiologist. You make me very nervous with that heart issue."

I nodded, and promised to call Dr. Levine's office that afternoon to have the paperwork sent over.

In June, we were ready to start the cycle. Dr. Ryley had my cardiology letter of approval. I was optimistic, and trying to stay positive. I was doing guided meditation, taking recommended herbs, and doing acupuncture once a week. I went in for ultrasounds every few mornings, and one morning heard an "uh oh," from the nurse.

"What?" I said.

"It looks like two of the eggs are getting big. Dr. Ryley may want to trigger that so we don't lose out on them. They look great."

"It's too early!" I said. "Only two eggs? What about the eight others?" She said she would call me later with the final decision.

She called me that evening. "Dr. Ryley wants you to take the trigger shot tonight. All the other eggs may be too immature, but these look great." I agreed, feeling disappointed but understanding the doctor knew best.

The shot that I would take at midnight would cause me to ovulate and would release the eggs. The doctors would put me under anesthesia and would then come in thirty-six hours later to retrieve the eggs and inject the sperm directly into the eggs in the lab. I prayed that this would work. The last two cycles we had gotten only one or two fertilized eggs from four or five released eggs, so this was very risky.

A few days later, I woke from the procedure with Andrew by my side. "Hon, don't get upset." He said, rubbing my hand. I braced myself for disappointment.

"What's wrong?" I cried.

"They got only one egg."

I clutched my chest. "Oh, my God! This is never going to work!" I began hyperventilating.

The nurse approached me and patted me on my shoulder. "Sweetie, it only takes one good egg. You have to stay positive."

I began to shake and cry, knowing this would not work. So many people had told me "it only takes one," and I felt like strangling anyone who said it. This whole IVF process had left me feeling angry, helpless, anxious, tired, impatient, and frustrated since we had begun.

I left the clinic a few hours later, trying to stay hopeful, but knowing my chances were slim. Andrew was keeping me sane, and encouraged me to stay hopeful.

The night before the transfer, Dr. Ryley called me. "I know you are feeling disappointed, Allison. I just wanted to let you know I saw the embryo, and it is flawless. I have a really great feeling about this one."

Chapter 7

The Psychic

THE DAY BEFORE THE TRANSFER, WE DECIDED TO take a day trip to Salem, Massachusetts. Many storefronts had signs for psychic readings, and though it was not something I generally believed in, we thought it would be fun.

The store we entered was filled with leather jackets and small trinkets, bath goods, and souvenirs. In the back was a small cave-like room with a dark drapery hanging over an open doorway for privacy. Andrew and I both thought this was a silly idea, but it was all in the spirit of hanging out in Salem.

Before I went in, Andrew whispered into my ear, "Don't say anything about IVF or pregnancy. Just see if she brings it up." I nodded, desperate for her to tell me good news. Andrew had different intentions for his session. He did not want to know anything about the future, as he claimed it made him nervous.

I decided to go in alone, because in my typical nature, the future was all I wanted to know about. After a few minutes of what I considered unimportant, albeit true monologue about my personality, the psychic said, "Allison, I hope you don't mind me saying this, but I see a dark cloud over your head, and I believe it has to do with babies."

I nodded.

"You were sick. Very sick. In the hospital for a while. A lot happened, and it has been tremendously difficult. You have had some help to get pregnant, but you had a few losses."

My eyes welled up. Though my losses were early, seeing a positive pregnancy test turn into negative only days to weeks later was devastating.

"Listen, this one is going to work. I'm seeing a boy. An Aquarius." She saw me counting on my hands. I knew if we got pregnant now, the baby would be due in April, not a February or March Aquarius. "He will be early, but he will be fine."

I nodded, knowing this was all baloney. She went on to tell me unimportant facts about my finances and social life, and I was on my way.

As Andrew and I sat down for lunch, I recounted what she had told me. "It was bizarre, like she knew everything I had been through, but it just doesn't make any sense. If the baby is an Aquarius, it would have to be two months early!" He shook his head, and we changed topics and enjoyed our lunch.

I went to the clinic the next day, did my acupuncture, and had the egg transferred into me. For the next three days, I put myself on self-imposed bed rest, getting up only to eat and sleep. Everyone had told me this was unnecessary, but I felt that I had continued my normal activities on the last three cycles, overdid it at times, and needed to let my body fully rest to make for a more hospitable environment for the embryo. I avoided the gym, ate well, and allowed myself plenty of couch and TV time. During the dreaded two week wait, we went out for dinner, saw a comedy show, and did a few day trips. I was trying to not obsess about the test, and the distraction was working.

I went in for my blood tests early one morning in July. My nephew Jacob had been born the week before my test; holding him in my arms at one day old made me realize the depth of my hope for a baby. I prayed and meditated daily for the cycle to work. That afternoon, I went to go visit my parents. I paced their living room, awaiting the call form the nurse.

"Allison?" she said. I was accustomed to a voice of pity on the other line, but her tone was positive and perky. "I have great news! Your test came back positive, and your numbers look great! Continue taking the progesterone, and come back in two days for a repeat test."

I started jumping up and down, as my mom hovered nearby. "That's awesome! Thanks so much!" My mom came over to embrace me. "I'm not getting too excited yet, Mom. This has happened before."

I was waiting to be devastated, so I only shared this news with Andrew, my parents, and my sister

Emily. Two days later, when the HCG had more than doubled, I allowed my excitement to grow. They wanted to see me one week later to check the HCG status. This was the highest it had been in all of the cycles. We continued to keep this secret until our eight-week ultrasound appointment, where it was confirmed there was indeed a strong heartbeat, and everything looked good thus far.

Chapter 8

The Pregnancy

I was terrified. This pregnancy felt too good to be true. I had no morning sickness and felt wonderful and energetic for the first few weeks. At the end of the day, I would be tired and a bit swollen, but I kept up with my yoga classes and daily walks. When I was cleared to begin teaching again, I returned to my former teaching schedule of daily fitness and yoga classes.

At ten weeks pregnant, I noticed that my face looked puffy. When I'd bend over, I felt a sense of suffocation, my face would turn beet red, and I couldn't take a breath. Downward facing dogs in yoga became torturous, and walking up our steep driveway would require resting on the porch stairs for minutes afterward. I gained weight at a rapid pace despite eating the same amount of healthy foods and watching my sodium as I was required to do.

I wanted to be that huge pregnant woman who practiced yoga until the day she went into labor, but I knew I would not be practicing for much longer. I took my search to Dr. Google, and all results came back telling me the blood volume increase is high while pregnant, causing many women to experience breathlessness and fluid retention.

By week twelve, I had gained twenty pounds. I made an appointment with Dr. Levine. I knew something was not right but said nothing to Andrew. He was already worrying about me, and I hated making his anxiety any worse.

"Your body is gaining as much as it needs to for the baby," My midwife told me. She had warned me early on that if anything seemed abnormal at all, I would need to consult with Dr. Economy, and I would be unable to do a natural, midwife-assisted birth.

I studied my natural birthing books and did guided visualizations to prepare for a natural labor. However, as I felt worse, I had a gut feeling that natural labor would not be my path. Dr. Levine told me to take more diuretics. They didn't help.

The first few weeks Andrew took a weekly belly shot photo, and I proudly stood sideways to show my nonexistent belly. Now looking back at the photos, I see the excitement and confidence gone from my eyes by week sixteen. I remember Andrew asking, "Ready to do the picture?" and feeling pained to get off the couch.

I no longer felt like a cute, pregnant lady; I felt fat and swollen. I was exhausted, out of breath, anxious about why I was gaining so much weight, and obsessed about what might be wrong with me. Not ready for a photo opportunity.

I had no appetite, yet could gain three pounds a day. Andrew would tell me how beautiful I was, and I felt guilty over my lack of enjoyment about the pregnancy. We had known we were having a boy, but it was hard to get excited when I was so positive that something was wrong.

When I woke one morning, I took the dog on a walk and came back with pain and swelling in my genitals. When I called Andrew to complain, I compared my vagina to two Twinkies.

"Maybe you should call Dr. Levine," Andrew said. "This is what happened in 2010 when you were fluid overloaded."

I pressed into my ankle and saw pitting, meaning my fingerprint indent stayed in place. I called Dr. Levine, who told me to take more diuretics, that I would keep having edema regardless, but the medication should keep it tolerable.

When I went in to see the midwife, she did an exam and said, "Wow. That looks really painful. I honestly think that is the worst vaginal swelling I have ever seen. It can happen sometimes."

"But why?" I cried, sitting up on the exam table, gathering my johnny around my legs.

"There is a lot of pressure pushing down there. I'll call in some prescription compression underpants."

I laughed when she told me that the compression would keep the swelling down, and that I could also ice the area. Although I joked about the situation with my friends, I knew what I was experiencing was not normal. I was in pain, and I was terrified.

As the days passed, Andrew was getting paranoid, so I tried to refrain from complaining to him. The reality was, my day consisted of walking the dog and having difficulty breathing, coming home to rest, and seeing clients while making sure both legs were elevated on an ottoman in my office. Fortunately, working at home allowed me to arrange my circumstances for added comfort. If my legs dangled from a chair, they would get painful, swollen and filled with fluid. I had to spend most of my days with my legs up.

I was still teaching my fitness and yoga classes; by this time, my students and clients knew I was pregnant. I did not have a big belly, but my overall appearance had changed so much with the swelling it was impossible to hide. I tried not to walk around during the classes, instead sitting and instructing from the front of the room.

"Hon, maybe you should take a break from teaching until after the baby comes," Andrew suggested one night while I picked over my dinner. I shook my head. I was not throwing in the towel yet. My body felt out of control, and I felt like I needed my normal structure and routine to keep any sense of normalcy.

I put my yoga membership on hold one day after taking a class with my friend Lauren. She was due at the same time I was and flowed through the class with no problem. I felt like a beached whale, and I could not breathe. I was only twenty weeks along. It was then that I knew I had to slow down and listen to my body. I'd gone to the same yoga studio almost daily. The owners Kevan and Betty had supported me on the whole IVF journey. They knew when I was cycling and helped me to modify accordingly. During my pregnancy, I had gotten emotional many times in class during practice. They provided me with endless compassion and support.

The following week, things progressed towards danger. My vagina was completely swollen, by body was about thirty-five pounds up, I couldn't move around without gasping for air, and I just wanted to sleep. My appetite was nonexistent. On Thursday, November 21, I vomited after eating a little yogurt and granola for dinner.

"I think I have the stomach flu, hon," I told Andrew. "Something is not right. I feel terrible."

I went to bed early but was unable to sleep. I felt nauseous and out of breath. I lay supported by three pillows, looking at the ceiling. I had slept in a seated position for weeks, as it was difficult to breathe when lying down.

At 1 a.m., I decided I could not wait until morning to talk to my OB/GYN. I shook Andrew awake.

"I can't sleep. I am going to the ER. Something is wrong. I think I have the stomach flu, or something is off. I may as well just go now, since I will have to deal with traffic in the morning. I want to make sure the baby is getting everything he needs."

"I'll go with you," he said, climbing out of bed.

"I'll be fine, hon. Don't worry. Go back to sleep. They'll probably just hydrate me and send me home. But I should get it checked out. I'll call you as soon as they tell me anything." I went downstairs and packed a backpack with my phone, wallet, bottle of water, and a book.

Chapter 9

The ER

As I pulled up to the ER at the local hospital, I parked my car in the temporary parking out front. I figured I wouldn't be there long and didn't feel like I could make the walk from the parking garage to the ER entrance. There was no wait, and a nurse took my history and information. When she asked about my cardiac history, she told me she needed to make a few calls. She asked for the specific diagnosis.

"Well, there never really was one," I replied. "It was in 2010, and the mass that had appeared in my right ventricle disappeared with steroids and a gluten free diet for my celiac disease." Her eyes widened as she nodded and disappeared from the room for a few minutes.

She came back with a gown. "We are going to send you in for an echocardiogram."

I shook my head. "My cardiologist has done one recently. It was fine! I am pretty sure I have a stomach bug. I can't seem to hold any food down, and I just don't feel great." She assured me this was protocol for anyone with a cardiac history, so I got dressed in the gown and followed her. After the echo, they took blood, put me in a room and told me to wait for the doctor.

I sent a text to my parents and siblings, telling them that I was sick with the stomach flu and was in the hospital, but I was doing fine. I waited a few more minutes for the doctor to arrive.

"Allison, we are going to send you over to the cardiology team at Brigham and Women's. There is an ambulance waiting outside for you."

"What? Why?" I cried.

"Your echo shows a significant problem with your heart's functioning right now. Your cardiac enzymes are also very high. The cardiology team there is better equipped to manage this."

I nodded my head, in shock. "Is the baby okay?" It was the only thing that mattered to me right then.

"There was a normal heartbeat detected on the ultrasound during the echo, but obviously your OB needs to take a look."

I burst out crying, and said, "I need to call my family!" I called Andrew and my parents, who all said they would meet me at the hospital when I arrived.

The next few hours were a haze of doctors, med students, nurses, and tests. I was panicked, demanding they ultrasound my belly to make sure the baby was safe. We had chosen to name the baby Ethan, after my Grandma Estelle. I was accustomed to this heart drama, but wondering if Ethan was okay made my want to throw my body on the hospital floor in a tantrum.

The ER room team admitted me to the cardiac floor where my family met me. Hooked up to a holter monitor and chest electrodes, I was able to talk to Dr. Economy as her tech did a bedside ultrasound.

Dr. Economy said, "Baby looks totally fine! Let's just wait to see what the cardiologists have to say. Seems like the blood volume changes from pregnancy flared up your heart condition."

I breathed a sigh of relief as I squeezed Andrew's hand. "See, hon? It's going to be fine! They'll just get some of these fluids off me and I'll be able to go home in a few hours."

Andrew gave me a doubtful look and said, "I think we need to wait to hear what they say. They may want to monitor you for a few days."

I was sure that due to my prior heart condition, my body was just taking on extra stress from the baby. The doctors would prescribe diuretics to get the fluid off. We had planned to go to Florida for our babymoon vacation in two weeks, and I felt confident I'd be home within hours.

The hours passed while we waited for answers.

"I think they are probably going to end up keeping me overnight," I said. "Hon, you should get home to walk the dog. Mom and Dad, I'll be fine. I'll call you if I hear anything."

A few minutes after my parents left, the attending doctor entered the room. I could not read her expression but started to prepare myself for a required bed rest. In my head, that was the worst-case scenario. I was prepared to follow whatever instructions she gave to keep Ethan healthy.

The next part of this story is hard for me to tell, since I believe I went into shock after hearing what the doctor told me.

"Allison, we have extensively gone over your records, and we feel confident that we know what is going on. The functioning of your right ventricle is extremely limited right now, and you are having pretty severe tricuspid regurgitation. This can explain why you gained so much weight so rapidly during this pregnancy. Your heart is in failure."

My jaw dropped, and I looked at Andrew's horrified face. This was not what I expected to hear. I couldn't react, and my body froze. I brought my hands to my belly as if to protect Ethan and cried, "What?"

"You have something called endomyocardial fibrosis. This is a condition in which the heart muscle slowly starts to get rigid and eventually stops working all together. Let me ask you a question, have you traveled to the tropics or South Africa recently?" I laughed, nervous, feeling as if I was watching this entire interaction from above.

Andrew answered for me. "No, Doctor, why?"

"Well, this condition is traditionally seen when someone picks up a parasite while traveling in these countries. Quite rarely, it happens as a result of an autoimmune disorder. It sounds like Allison is one of these rare cases. We have never seen this condition at this hospital, so to be honest, I would like to do a little more research before we decide what to do. The entire team will need to meet, and we will come up with a treatment plan." I nodded my head.

"The baby will be okay, right?" I asked. I gave Andrew a nervous glance.

"Right now, we need to make sure you are safe. We are going to admit you for observation and start you on IV lasiks to get some of the fluids off. I will say this. I know this is going to come as a shock to you, Allison, but people with this condition eventually need a heart transplant. There is no way to know in how many months or years, but you will need a new heart."

My stomach dropped to my feet, as I feared I would vomit. I was sitting on the edge of a stiff white bed, my back facing the doorway to my room. My legs dangled down and I stared at my swollen bare feet. I swallowed, tearing welling in my eyes. I hated this doctor with a passion and wanted her out of my room.

"Thank you, I am done," I said, numb. She tried to touch my shoulder and I shrugged her off. "That's all, thank you." I couldn't let myself get upset. I knew she was wrong, and I just wanted her to leave my room. I was a thirty-one-year-old woman who ate healthy foods, exercised daily, wore sun block, didn't smoke or drink, had never done drugs. There was no way I was in heart failure. A heart transplant?

She began to talk again. Her lips moved, but I had no idea what she was saying. I kept my back to her and focused on the lights of the city outside my window. I complained about the cold the day before, but in that moment I would have given anything to be out there and not in the hospital. As if in slow motion, I looked around the room in disbelief, wishing my parents were still there and that my poor anxious husband had not been here to hear this news. I felt constant guilt about how he already worried about me, and I knew this might push him over the edge.

"Thank you, doctor. I'm done now." I curled up in a ball in the bed and turned my back to her.

Andrew said, "I think she has had enough for tonight. Thank you, Doctor. I think she just needs to rest."

The doctor left the room, and I began to hyperventilate. "I hate her!" I screamed to Andrew. "I never want to see her again! She's fucking crazy! I don't need a heart transplant. This is a bad dream!" My body shook, and Andrew tried to calm me down and hold me. "No! This is a bad dream! What the fuck? I just want to go home. Why does everything need to be such a battle? I can't breathe. I need something. I can't breathe."

A nurse rushed in after Andrew hit the call button, and then left to come back with a shot of ativan to calm me down. After about twenty minutes, I passed out on my bed. I woke up the next morning, confused as to what had happened the night before.

Chapter 10

Life in the Hospital

I HEARD THE BIG SCALE ROLLING DOWN THE HALL toward my room each morning at 6 a.m. At twenty-one weeks pregnant, I feared that every pound of weight gain meant my heart was going to stop, and Ethan and I could both die. Every day my weight lowered, I felt more energetic and healthy. After four days in the Shapiro Center, I had lost thirty pounds of fluids while on IV diuretics and was lower than my pre-pregnancy weight.

I anticipated our "big meeting" with the cardiovascular and Ob/GYN teams. The potential heart transplant had not been brought up again; I wanted to pretend I imagined it. Now that the water weight was coming off, and I was feeling so well, I thought the worst case scenario would be going on home bed rest for the remainder of the pregnancy. I told some close friends that I was in the hospital and word began to spread. I assured everyone that it was a scare, and we would be home in a few days.

I had not heard from Dr. Levine, but my family was furious that he had given me medical clearance to get pregnant. The day before Thanksgiving, I saw his office number on my caller ID. In shock, I decided to let the phone go to voice mail.

"Hi Allison, it's Dr. Levine. I know you must be very angry with me, and I wanted to let you know I am thinking of you and hope you are feeling okay. I hope you can try to have a nice, salt-free Thanksgiving." In the voice mail, he chuckled, sounding nervous. It took every ounce of will power not to throw my phone at a wall. I was livid.

It was obvious to me that my new doctors, without directly criticizing another physician, thought Dr. Levine had made a big mistake in approving pregnancy. He had missed a major, life-threatening diagnosis. Dr. Levine had told me I had an enlarged right ventricle, when the new doctors found the ventricle to be tiny and constricted, with the atrium enlarged. My heart was beating at a limited capacity, with only a third of the heart muscle working.

I decided to not focus on my anger about the misdiagnosis. After all, if I had come to Brigham in the first place, I would never have been cleared to be pregnant. I was scared for our lives, but my sick heart felt attached to Ethan, and I was not going to give up on him.

Chapter 11

The Meeting

THE DOCTORS WERE READY TO SEE US. ANDREW was on his way from work. I had waited all day, and we were called into the family meeting room at the end of the hallway at 6 p.m. Andrew had started a new job the week that I was hospitalized, and I wanted to ensure that my hospitalization would not jeopardize his new career. He traveled to and from the hospital after work, stopping at home to walk our dog, Maddie. I felt a tremendous amount of guilt for the hospitalization and how stressed it made Andrew.

Before we decided to get pregnant, he had questioned the cardiologist multiple times if I would be safe while pregnant. It was as if he knew in his gut that I would not be. Given that Andrew is a self-proclaimed hypochondriac, this whole hospitalization was his worst nightmare come true.

We decided to start the meeting with Andrew on speakerphone in the car. My parents held my arm as we walked down the long hallway, wheeling my IV pole along. I looked into the other patients' rooms as we walked, most of them elderly and lying in their beds all day. I was the only young person on the floor. As I walked the hall, I could look up on the nurses' screens, and see what my heart was doing. My resting heart rate was about 130; walking would make it soar.

My siblings Dan and Emily waited for us in the family room. Andrew's mom Ellen had driven down from Vermont to be at the meeting. I took a seat near the door, my favorite beige fake leather lounge chair that would allow me to kick my feet up and lean back. The room was packed with doctors, residents, and a few nurses sitting on the couches and all staring at me with what I interpreted as pity. My armpits began to sweat, and I scratched the dry skin on my arms while I waited for someone to talk. I mentally reminded myself to apply more coconut oil to my arms after the meeting was over with.

Dr. Economy began. "Allison, we have reviewed all of the medical history and the current echocardiograms. As you know, you have a serious condition called endomyocardial fibrosis. We believe that the stress on the heart caused by the pregnancy is ultimately going to cause your heart to fail." I sat up straighter in my chair, my attention focused on Dr. Economy. I fiddled with the IV pole next to my body, pumping magnesium and potassium into my bloodstream. I glanced around the room and noticed everyone staring at me intensely. I felt a dissociation, as if I were watching someone in a movie scene.

"I know this is a very difficult decision," Dr. Economy continued, "but we think that for your safety, you cannot remain pregnant. It is just too risky. Both you and the baby could die. We know you love your baby, but I'm sure all of the people in the room would rather keep you alive than have both of you not make it through this."

Tears were streaming down my face. My brain raced with panic and fury. I thought about the baby toys, the crib, the stroller, and the clothes, all of it sitting upstairs in the nursery at home.

I thought about the IVF treatments, the tears, the frustration, and finally the elation with the positive pregnancy test. Ethan was a part of my heart and soul. I was not ready to give him up because of a maybe.

"No." I stated. I knew I would not change my mind. Nothing that anyone said could have made me change my mind. I noticed some eyes shifting, glances around the room, and tears from my family.

"We are not asking you to make up your mind right now, Ali." Dr. Economy said.

"No." I started to get agitated. "No! Ethan is perfect and has had no health issues. No. We worked too hard to get pregnant, and I am not giving up on this baby. No."

My dad's face was red, and I knew he was getting angry with me. My mother-in-law Ellen's eyes were welling up with tears.

"Ali, you have to listen to the doctors," my brother Dan said.

My dad wouldn't look at me, instead gave a knowing and nervous look to my mother, then numbly gazed out the window at the Boston traffic. We both knew that I was going to continue saying no. It was in my blood—my stubborn determination and eternal optimism. Dad considered himself a realist, although I thought of him as a pessimist. As a retired physician, he knew the enormity of what I was refusing to do.

"I will not abort Ethan. I can feel him kicking and moving inside me every day. Maybe it is easy for all of you because he doesn't feel real to you, but he is very real to me. I'm done with this meeting." I started to stand so I could walk back to my room.

Ellen got down on her knees next to me, sobbing. "You can't do this to Andrew, Ali! You just can't! You have to save yourself!"

My eyes teared up again in frustration and anger. What about what I wanted? What about the baby?

Dr. Nohria, the attending doctor who had originally given me my diagnosis, took over. "Ali, you have had this condition for years. It was missed by your other doctors because the condition is so rare. If you had come to me with this diagnosis, I would have told you that you could never be pregnant, and to pursue alternative options like adoption or surrogacy. We received your records from your old doctor, and all the echocardiograms tell us the same story. You could die if you decide to stay pregnant. The likelihood is that you both will die. Or we would need to place you on a machine to make your heart work, and the baby *still* could die. You have enough time before the baby is viable at twenty-four weeks to have an abortion. And your family and doctors will be here to support you and take the next step."

"No. I said I was done. Thank you. If my heart starts failing in the next few days, maybe things will change. But I feel great now that the fluid is off, and I just won't do it."

The doctors nodded at one another. One of them said, "We will leave you to discuss this with your family."

My brother Dan got out of his chair. I could tell he was furious. "Ali, if you don't listen to the doctors, I won't support this decision at all. I'm not fucking supporting this pregnancy. I won't visit you, and I won't have anything to do with it. I came here directly from my friend's wake, and they gave us these." He tossed a prayer card into my lap from the service. "I'm not making one of these for your funeral." And with that, he left.

I sat in my chair with my knees folded up to my chest. My mouth hung open, and I felt numb. I had no idea that Dan had been at a wake, but I let that thought pass as I stared at my legs in front of me. I thought about how thin my legs looked now that the fluid was off, and that I did not really look pregnant anymore. I was getting used to my lack of belly again, as much of the fluid was retained in that area.

My sister Emily stood up and walked over to me. She bent down to my level, took my shoulders and locked eyes with me. At that point, Andrew was walking in the door. He had tears in his eyes, and I had to look away. He had heard it all on conference call. He watched me while Emily spoke.

"Listen to me, Ali. I love you and I'm going to support you. I know you really want Ethan, but we all want you alive! I will still support you no matter what you decide to do."

I gave my sister a hug, and said, "Thanks, pook. Love you. I've already made up my mind."

"I know," she said. I trusted my gut, but at the same time felt that something catastrophic may happen and perhaps I had spoken too soon.

My parents stood and left the room. On the way out my mother said, "I'll call you tomorrow." My dad ignored me. Both of them were crying.

Andrew walked over to me, took me in his arms, and I began to hyperventilate again. We walked out of the room and down the hall with my IV dragging behind. When we got to my room, I fell apart. I lay down on the bed and began moaning and sobbing. "Why is this happening? I don't understand. I can't take this anymore!"

Andrew held me and tried to reassure me. I couldn't stop crying, and a nurse came in to give me medications to calm me down.

Months later, Andrew told me that everyone in the family was calling him over those next few days to tell him how he needed to convince me to abort Ethan. He told me how much he struggled with wanting the baby but also felt terrified of losing me in my passion to become a mother. He felt a tremendous weight on his shoulders; pressure put on him by both of our families—that he didn't love me enough to tell me to have an abortion.

Chapter 12

Pregnant Life

THE NEXT FEW DAYS MOVED AT A SLOW PACE. Everyone danced around the topic of abortion. I felt great, looked much better and less puffy, and was feeling optimistic. I had an ultrasound, and the doctors told me the baby looked great. I spent my days reading books and magazines, watching TV shows that I would never allow myself to watch under normal circumstances, engaging in phone sessions with clients, and having friends and family visit.

My brother came in with his wife Holly and their son Jacob. He took me aside and hugged me. He said, "When I got home that night, Holly talked some sense into me. She told me she would have done the same with Jake, and that really gave me some perspective on the whole thing. I love you, and I'm sorry for saying what I did."

He later told me that he was the one who got my parents on board with my decision. They visited me daily, but they would not make eye contact or talk more than short sentences related to bringing food or clothing. I knew what they wanted me to do, and

I would not agree to it. My parents know that one of my best and worst qualities is my persistence. When I make up my mind about something, I am stubborn about getting my way. I was like that as a child, and it hasn't changed to this day.

At twenty-two weeks pregnant, the family and my doctors held another meeting. Everyone sat around my bedside while I took a painful potassium infusion in my IV. I was in the middle of eating eggs, and I was frustrated that I had no sense of privacy in this room. Anyone could walk in whenever they wanted.

The message was: "We understand that you are going to keep the pregnancy, Ali. Our goal is to keep you as healthy as we can. But as soon as we see any signs of acute heart failure, our plan is to induce labor, whether or not we think the baby will make it. Your OB team can focus on the baby, but our primary goal is to keep you alive."

I had been able to select one of my favorite doctors, Dr. Neal Lakdawala to lead my case. I trusted and respected him. He had toddler twins, and I felt as if he understood and supported my decision. I nodded my head, eager for the abortion discussion to end.

Back at home, word was getting out around the community. Before the hospitalization, I was teaching multiple fitness and yoga classes each week. I decided to update my students, friends, and family on Facebook to put various circulating rumors to rest. The owners and teachers from my yoga studio asked if it would be okay to hold a class in my honor that week. I felt embarrassed to be getting the attention, and unworthy since I had convinced myself at that point that I was fine. I believed I would not need a heart transplant, and I would heal after the baby came. I thought I might eventually need one, but that so many advances in medical technology would come within the next few years that there would soon be some less invasive option, or perhaps some new medication.

All the same, I told Kevan, Betty and Becca from my yoga studio that I would be honored, and that I wish I could practice with them. I missed yoga! When I had quit practicing at twenty weeks, I had no clue that my feelings of suffocation were due to the heart failure, and that I would not return to a yoga class for about a year after that.

In the following days, Sarah, a friend of mine who runs a charity called "Yoga Reaches Out" contacted me to see if she could create a "Rally for Ali" day, in which studios around New England would dedicate their practices to me, and raise funds for medical treatment.

At that point, my doctors were discussing the possibility of moving temporarily to another state for the transplant after the baby was born. The waiting lists for transplants in New England were the worst in the country. Due to the nature of my disease, I was not eligible for a ventricular assist device (VAD). My right ventricle was constricted and "too tiny." Doctors feared I would not make it without either one of these machines or a surgery. I was confident there would be an alternative surgery to fix my problem. I was even compiling scientific studies on various procedures that had been done to help endomyocardial fibrosis. Most studies indicated the patient would eventually be transplanted, but I chose to ignore those parts of the studies.

But somewhere in the back of my mind, I knew things could get bad, so I thanked Sarah for the idea and that I was touched by the idea. I thought the money raised could help pay for parking, meals, dog walking, and such for our family.

A few days later, I was shocked to see that Stil Studio and "Rally for Ali" raised over $10,000, which eventually helped us to fund most expenses and travel for my transplant. It amazed me how involved people became and how much they cared, and I still cannot thank everyone enough. I will never forget how much support and love my community showed for my family and the baby.

In my daily life at the hospital, I struggled with the lack of movement and with being stuck in a room all day. I tried to create a routine for myself, as I woke up each morning to the sounds of the huge scale rolling down the hallway. I was terrified to gain weight in fear of acute heart failure. At the same time, I was supposed to be gaining weight for the pregnancy and felt conflicted and confused when I stood on the scale every day.

A nurse technician would take my vital signs, and then I would be up and getting my tea ready. At twenty-three weeks I became extremely adverse to the smell and taste of coffee, so I had switched to tea. I would then do my "morning walk" where I would get my Ipod, put my sneakers on with my hospital gown, and do ten full walking laps around the hall. This would take about thirty minutes. My nurses would praise me for my dedication to my walking, as I tried to stay active and get up and move several times a day.

When I visit the floor now and breeze down the hallways, I remember how long it would take me to do those ten laps, how long I needed to lie down to rest afterwards. I got so used to compensating for so many years on a broken heart that I had gotten used to everything feeling challenging. In my boot camp classes, my students used to tease me when my lips turned purple. It would happen every time I did pushups or planks, and it was just "an Ali thing". Since I love to move and exercise, stopping wasn't even a question. I figured things were harder for me because I didn't have a 100 percent healthy heart, but I was fine. I trusted Dr. Levine to tell me otherwise. I did notice that if I completed a hard workout, I would be swollen and would gain five to ten pounds by the next morning, but tried not to obsess about it.

I remember the day I threw my scale away because I convinced myself I would always fluctuate, and it wasn't worth the stress anymore.

I was never one who was good at "being lazy" or sitting still all day, so this was the most challenging part of being in the hospital. My wonderful nurses moved me to the "Shapiro suite," the best room on the floor. I had a bedroom with a view overlooking Boston and a sitting room with a little kitchenette where I could sit with visitors. My nurses made me feel like I was living in a sorority house: Chrissie, Marie, Sherie, Amy, Jill, Katherine, Jackie, Morgan, Ashley, Wylie, Claire, Alyson, Heather, Debbie, Karen, Gretchen, Mary, Danielle, and Ally. They all felt like sisters to me and did their best to keep me happy and entertained. They comforted me when I was feeling sad or sorry for myself, and made the whole experience as pleasant as it could possibly be.

Emily came and decorated my room with Christmas lights, and we hung pictures to make it feel like home. But it wasn't home. Many of my friends were pregnant and due at the same time as Ethan. They would come visit, and we would giggle and gossip for hours. After they left, I would crawl in my uncomfortable hospital bed and sob. It felt unfair that everyone I knew seemed to have a healthy and easy pregnancy.

They were able go home and live normal lives after they visited me. I imagined them saying to their husbands, "Man, I feel so bad for Ali. That would suck to be stuck in that room all day and pregnant."

I wanted to get "pregnant lady attention"—people touching my belly and asking when I was due. Instead, I was getting the sick girl attention, a role I had gotten used to since dealing with my first heart scare in 2010. I was tired of being the sick girl.

In the first few weeks, the doctors told me they were amazed by how well I was doing. They decided to let me go downstairs to the café with my parents one afternoon. I was feeling good while going down, but started to get woozy while in the café, drinking an iced tea.

I interrupted my dad. "Um, I think I need to go back upstairs now. I just don't feel great." He grabbed my arm and helped me up, and I felt my knees weaken as we got closer to the elevator.

Before I knew what was happening, my knees buckled and my dad started yelling, "Code blue! Code blue!" In that moment, I thought this was it. I was dying. Maybe I actually wasn't going to make it through this. I should have just listened to the doctors about ending the pregnancy.

When we got back upstairs, they tested my blood sugar and told me it was at fifty, which is why I almost fainted. I made a mental note to eat more food more often. My dad teases me now that when I went down that day, I still managed to hold my iced tea up so it would not spill.

In the weeks leading up to the hospitalization, I had gained about thirty pounds very rapidly, and I panicked that I was doing something wrong, or that I was going to give my kid diabetes. I was not "eating for two" but couldn't help but feel terrible about my weight gain and my body being out of control. After my collapse, I realized that I had actually gained almost no weight during this pregnancy. I needed to push past food aversions and lack of appetite to get some good quality food in my body.

Since I was going to be in the hospital for months, the social workers arranged for someone to shop for me weekly at Whole Foods. I kept getting sick from cross contamination of gluten in the prepared cafeteria foods.

Andrew would joke, "You'll never want to come home after this royal treatment!" The truth was that I missed our home life more than ever. I would face time with Andrew after he left the hospital every night, and then cry myself to sleep. I just wanted to watch a movie while snuggling with my husband on our couch.

Weeks passed, and I had good days and bad. At twenty-four weeks, the Ob/GYN wanted to give me one more chance to make a decision by showing me what the babies in the NICU looked like. I had purchased several books about preemies from Amazon, and knew that Ethan could be very sick if he was born at twenty-four weeks. I refused to go to the NICU until I started feeling like he was closer to being born. Once the water weight was off, I looked healthy, vibrant, and was full of positive thoughts and energy. I knew my heart had more potential without the edema, and I was confident that I would go past twenty-four weeks. The doctors were mentioning twenty-eight weeks as a final cutoff for when they would induce, as they were convinced that each passing week put my heart at greater risk to go into sudden failure.

At twenty-eight weeks, I still felt great. I agreed to visit the NICU to take a tour. Katherine, one of my favorite nurses, took me. She held my hand as I sobbed while talking with the NICU charge nurse about the complications that many preemies had. Katherine pushed me in a wheelchair through the rows of babies who were the size of my finger, and babies who were on breathing machines, tubes, and nestled in shoebox like incubators. Tears rolled down my face as I clenched the blanket in my lap and Katherine squeezed my shoulders. I felt like a tremendous failure as a mom, that I would be exposing my son to this world earlier than he needed to be here, simply because of my sick heart. I left the NICU with Katherine pushing me back to Shapiro, feeling deflated and defeated.

Thanks to my nurses, every day passed quickly. My parents came to visit me daily, along with Andrew most evenings, my siblings after work and on weekends when they could, and my wonderful friends. We celebrated holidays together in my hospital living room; first Thanksgiving, followed by Chanukah, Christmas, and New Year's. The doctors could not believe how well I was doing with the IV diuretics.

One afternoon, Dr. Economy came in with her colleagues Dr. Smith and Dr. Little, while Andrew and I were watching a movie. They gathered around my bed, looking down at me.

"Ali, we are so happy with how well you are doing. We have decided we are not going to set a cut off of twenty-eight weeks. We are just going to follow you closely. There actually is a chance you could get to thirty weeks or so! The longer you can keep that baby in there, the less time he will need in the NICU."

I looked at Andrew's face as it fell. I knew that he felt each day I was pregnant, the worse my chances were of staying alive and healthy.

"Are you sure that's a good idea, Dr. E?" Andrew asked. "Haven't we pushed our luck already? Why don't we just induce while she is healthy?"

"Andrew, like I said, Allison is doing great, and so is Ethan. As long as she is healthy and can keep that baby in there, the healthier the baby will be. I promise, the team is keeping a close eye on her. If anything starts to seem dangerous, we are going to induce."

Chapter 13

Reality Hits

THE NEXT DAY, I WAS WAITING FOR MY PARENTS to come visit when the social worker came into the room and asked me to sit down.

She said, "Ali, the team has decided to start your transplant evaluation. We want to get the ball rolling for you to get listed as soon as you have Ethan."

"What? Why?" I said. "I am doing great! What if I don't need a transplant?"

She patted my leg, "Ali, the doctors think that even though you are doing great, you are definitely going to need a transplant at some point in the next few years. You can't be listed now, but when you have the baby you can be. It is just easier to do this now and have it done with and ready."

I started crying. "This is so dumb. I don't need a transplant."

She assured me it would only take a few days. I would need to have meetings with different teams including psychiatry, social work, nutrition, pharmacology, general cardiology, infectious diseases, and finances. I rolled my eyes in frustration, knowing I had no choice.

My cardiologist had talked to us about possibly moving after I had the baby, so that I could get a heart faster than I would in New England. My father had done some research and found that Tampa General Hospital had good reviews and performed over fifty transplants per year. I was still in denial about moving or needing the surgery, so I had thanked my father but told him his research was unnecessary at this point. I was beginning to think I might be wrong.

I called my dad, crying. "They are insisting on doing this whole thing today and tomorrow! I don't get it! They don't even know that I need it. Why put me through all of this?"

My dad asked if I wanted him to talk to someone to put it on hold. I told him no, that I decided to go ahead and get it over with.

I began the evaluation with a curt and unpleasant psychiatrist, who did her interview with no emotion or empathy for my tears or the trauma I was experiencing. I spent the rest of the next two days miserable and angry at the world, refusing visits from anyone. Christmas was coming, and so was the snow. I was alone, tired, depressed, and feeling sorry for myself. I told Andrew that he should go to Vermont to celebrate Christmas with his family.

I often wondered if Andrew would have been happier if he hadn't married me. I felt like I was such a burden to him. I caused him worry, and he always had to take care of me. He was a self-described anxious worrywart, and this heart situation had turned his world upside down. I wanted him to experience normalcy and have fun during the holidays. He argued with me, but I convinced him to go.

I spent the holiday snuggled under my covers watching Christmas movies and looking out into the snowy Boston scenery. I reflected on why I had pushed him away, and realized it was because I was tired of feeling guilty. When I had visitors, I was thrilled to have the company, but felt terrible that they had to take the time out of their schedule to come to the hospital. My parents were both creatures of habit, and I knew that I was wrecking their daily routine. They cancelled their vacation to Florida in January, and I hated myself for that. There would never be enough apologies in the world for how much I had stressed out my family; those thoughts went through my mind constantly. On one hand, I was happy to have the support from family and friends. On the other hand, I wished I were alone, because the guilt of stressing others out made me feel horrible.

I got through the holidays and New Year's, and began to grow impatient with living in the hospital. The days were long and cold, and the frequent snow storms canceled planned visits that I looked forward to. My wonderful nurses would come in to chat with me and make sure I was happy, but I was lonely and very homesick.

Still, I wanted to stay pregnant for as long as possible so Ethan could grow bigger and more stable. At twenty-four weeks, they had given me a steroid shot to help his lungs develop faster, and I would get another shot once they decided to induce me. It was a waiting game at this point. When would my heart give out, and when would they need to get Ethan?

The morning of January 31, I had been in the hospital over two months when Dr. Economy came in and told me she had good news. "We have talked with the cardiology team, and since you are doing so well, we are going to let you carry this pregnancy as long as you can. That means Ethan may not even need the NICU, and you could possibly go full term."

I felt elated but frustrated. I was tired of the hospital and ready to go home. I knew it was the best for Ethan to grow to full term, but I also knew that the bigger he was, the harder the labor would be for me and for my heart. I was scared to die during labor, and I know that was what Andrew feared the most. The doctors had decided that a c-section would be far riskier for me, since the IV fluids would be more stressful for my heart. The goal was a vaginal birth, without letting me push. The doctors would use a vacuum to help me. I thanked Dr. Economy, and after she left I called my dad and Andrew on a group call.

Both were furious. "This is getting ridiculous," Andrew said. "We have pushed our luck. It's time to induce you! You are thirty-one weeks and he will do great. We should have induced at twenty-eight weeks. Any more than that and you are looking at a riskier birth for you!"

My dad agreed. "We need to hold a meeting. This is just getting silly. We need an end date before something bad happens."

I nodded my head and decided to ask the cardiac team for a meeting the next day when they came to see me in rounds. Andrew was coming in later for a visit, so I decided to take my evening laps before he came. My back was starting to cramp, and I was not feeling great. My belly was growing enough to cause discomfort. I blamed the pain on the lack of sleep from the night before, and the lousy bed that made it impossible for me to sleep comfortably.

Andrew and I had a short visit that night, since he was going out to dinner with an old high school friend. I wanted to encourage him to keep his fun activities in place, since distraction tended to work well for him. I wanted him to live a normal life despite what was happening to us. He left at around seven, and I ordered my dinner; the same one I ordered every single night: shrimp and scallops over a garden salad with a hard-boiled egg, a side of fruit, and butternut squash puree. I decided after dinner to watch a movie and go to sleep early.

Chapter 14

Surprise!

EVERY MORNING I WOKE AT 3:30 A.M. ON THE dot, needing a snack, a drink, and a trip to the bathroom. On the morning of February 1, I used the bed rail to sit up so I could start my daily morning ritual. As I pulled myself up, I noticed I trickled out a little urine. I chuckled to myself and rolled my eyes. I was already peeing my pants, and I was only thirty-one weeks pregnant. I sat up, and when I put my feet on the ground, I heard a pop, and an explosion of water erupted out of me.

"Umm, Ashley?" I yelled for my nurse. "Ashley!" She came running into my room, eyes wide open when she saw the puddle of water on the floor.

"I think my water broke!" I said. More water came out of me as I walked towards the bathroom. "Yup. It definitely broke," I said, nervously giggling and standing in a huge puddle. Her eyes widened, and she paged the doctor.

Several nurses and techs came running into the room to help clean up and move me to the labor and delivery floor. As they rolled me down the hallway,

I called Andrew. "Hon, my water broke! Can you come?" Andrew was groggy and still half asleep, but sprang into action and told me he was on his way.

The cardiologists had a plan. When I went into acute failure, they would give me the medications to induce labor. The attending cardiologist would be there along with the heart surgeons, in case an emergency occurred. My nurses in Shapiro took me in a stretcher to labor and delivery. The team decided to give me another steroid shot to help develop the baby's lungs. I was transferred to a tiny room in labor and delivery. I looked around and felt grateful that I'd been living in Shapiro and not here. The bed filled up most of the room, and I could almost reach out and touch the walls with my arms. I felt relieved that we had made it to thirty-one weeks and confident that Ethan would be fine.

Dr. Smith was on call. I remembered meeting her several times, and really liked her calm demeanor, compared to many of my cardiologists' apparent state of panic during the pregnancy. When she checked me, she told me I was only 1 cm. dilated and about 50% effaced. "In other words," she said, "this could take a while. If you aren't progressing by tomorrow, we'll give you the medications to move this along. And we will also give the epidural, because we want this to be the least amount of stress on your body as possible." She started me on an IV of magnesium to delay the labor so that the steroids could help Ethan's lungs develop before I gave birth. The magnesium made my body get uncomfortably hot, and I felt nauseous and miserable. I was assured this was normal. She let the cardiology team know I was transferred to the Women's center, and told them she would keep them updated, but that my vital signs were stable, and it could take a few days here.

We decided to wait until first thing in the morning to call my family, since we thought it would be about forty-eight hours until the actual birth. My parents and sister came, and we played trivia and board games throughout my contractions. We laughed as we played a Saved by the Bell game, despite my contractions getting closer together. Some of them were rather painful, but I was experiencing them all in my lower back. As the day went on, I got exhausted and hungry. They asked me to not eat solid foods before the labor, so I started to decline. At about 6 p.m., my parents left to go home. My sister was hoping to stay for the labor, as we had decided she would be in the room. We asked Dr. Smith to check to see how dilated I was, and by 8 p.m., I was dilated only three centimeters.

"You should just go home, Em. This is going to be a long night," I said to my sister. I was squeezing Andrew's hand during a painful contraction in my back. I asked my nurse if I could get in a hot shower, since I had read that could help relieve some of the intensity of the contractions. She agreed.

Emily left, and Andrew picked up the paper to read while I got in the shower. The contractions were getting closer and more intense. I got in the shower and let the hot water hit my back while I sat on a stool, wincing each time a new contraction came. After about twenty minutes, I asked Andrew to help me get out. He came in with a towel and helped me get back into my gown. He brought me over to the large physioball that the nurse brought in for me. I sat on the ball, facing the bed, and he stood behind me rubbing my back.

"Let's try to get some sleep, hon," I said, although we both knew we would not be sleeping. The nurse had pulled out a "couch" for Andrew, which looked and felt like a padded table.

"I don't think either one of us is going to be getting much sleep," he said. We flipped the lights off and laid down to rest.

I could not sleep. A contraction was coming what felt like every other minute. I looked at the clock at around three am. Three o'clock was Ethan's golden hour. Every morning, like clockwork, I would wake from a deep sleep and need to get up to use the bathroom and have a snack. My water had broken at three. And now, here it was twenty-four hours later, at 3 a.m., and I felt an intense need go poop. I remembered the week before giggling with my nurse Chrissie as she told me about embarrassing labor stories, and that urgency she felt right before her babies were born.

I woke up Andrew. "Hon, I feel such a pressure down there. I think he's coming!" We called in the nurse.

"I don't think so, honey," she said. "You were only three cm a few hours ago."

"Can you call the doctor? I really feel something down there!"

A few minutes later, Dr. Smith swooped into the room with her calm demeanor. An anesthesiologist was by her side. "Why don't we go ahead and give you the epidural to help you get some rest. We also want to place an arterial line to keep your heart closely monitored during the labor once the cardiology team comes in." I nodded my head, and then experienced the most pain thus far while a student fiddled with my wrist trying to get a line into my artery. The doctor took over and asked me to turn on my side so he could administer the epidural in my back. He started to do so, and I let out a yell. "Someone needs to check me down there! I think I feel his head!"

Sure enough, when Dr. Smith opened up my gown to check, she said, "Let's move it."

At that point, I froze and was struck by sudden terror. I thought maybe they all had been right. There was a chance I could go into that room alive and die on the table. There was a chance something could be wrong with Ethan, or he wouldn't make it. There was a chance he could make it but I wouldn't, and Andrew would need to raise him on his own.

This was it. I began to moan and cry. We rolled into the room, it was mayhem. There were about twenty nurses and doctors running in opposite directions, clearly in a panic. The cardiology team had been called, but no one had arrived yet. My eyes widened in fear. The environment was overwhelming, and I couldn't catch my breath.

Dr. Smith saw the look in my eyes, and let out a loud whistle. Everyone stopped talking and moving. She said, "Everyone needs to take a deep breath and calm down. Let's stay positive and keep Ali nice and calm!" Then she leaned over and got directly in my face.

"I can't do this," I cried. "I just can't."

She grabbed my hand. "Listen to me. Listen," she said sternly. "You've got this. I know you do. You are strong. Use your yoga breath. You've gotten through all these months here. Ali, you can do this! You have to do this."

I looked at Andrew and saw tears in his eyes. I was ready to go. He stood by my side. I was waiting for Dr. Smith to get the forceps and the vacuum, but she stood at my straddled legs in the air and said, "Honey, he is ready to come! I need a few pushes, and he will be here."

I mustered up all the strength I had and pushed as hard as I could. I felt like a watermelon was being ripped out of me. I was scared if I pushed too hard, my heart would just stop, but I would not give up at this point.

And then I heard crying. Andrew was standing at my feet, sobbing, and I saw a tiny little creature being pulled out of me. It was the most incredible, indescribable moment of my life. Everything stopped: the noise, the people, the fear and panic. I heard my baby cry. He was pink and screaming, and the tears streamed from my face. "Is he ok?" I cried.

"He is perfect!" Dr. Smith held my hand. "Listen to that big cry! They are just going to check him out." I saw Ethan on a table ten feet away, Andrew standing over him taking photos while they wrapped him up. A nurse brought him over to me and placed him on my chest. There is no way to say this that does not sound cliché, but I immediately fell in love. My world changed in that one moment. He was pure joy, love, and miracle.

"What's his name?" the nurse said.

"Ethan Matthew," I said. "It means strong gift from God."

Chapter 16

We Made It!

HE WAS TINY, JUST ABOUT THE SIZE OF MY OPEN hand. Three pounds one ounce, measuring sixteen and a half inches. Ethan stopped crying the moment he was placed on my chest. I gazed down at him, happy tears pouring down my face.

Andrew and I took photographs, squealing with delight. My glasses were held together by a piece of white tape, after I had broken them in half while mashing my face into the bed during one particularly painful contraction. The emotional and physical pain of everything that had happened during the pregnancy was forgotten. All I knew was that I was put on earth to be Ethan's mother. No doctor could have stopped me. His life became more important than mine the moment I heard his heartbeat. Seeing his face had confirmed that my decision to ignore everyone's advice had been correct. I felt giddy, overwhelmed, and was completely in love with my little Ethan.

After the doctors had delivered my placenta, they rolled a plastic incubator over to us. "We are going to bring Ethan to the NICU for observation. Allison, the team will bring you to the ICU for your observation. This happened so much faster than we thought it would, so that's why no one made it in time! You'll need to lie flat for about thirty-six hours because of the fluid shifts. You need to be closely monitored by the nurses and doctors there."

I looked around the room. Nurses were cleaning up, and the doctors were talking in the corner. None of the cardiologists had made it to the delivery. I was in awe. The whole plan of inducing, me not pushing, and my potential of death during labor all had dissipated. I felt almost abandoned by my team, but knew once I felt that need to push and they realized Ethan was coming, it was impossible for the doctor on call to make it on time.

"Andrew can go with Ethan or with you," the doctor added.

"I'm fine," I said, without a second thought. "I want him to go with Ethan."

About an hour later, I lay in an ICU bed specifically measured at a forty-five degree angle. I asked a nurse to hand me the phone. I called the hospital operator and asked for the hospital lactation consultant. I wanted to feed Ethan. I did not want him getting formula in the NICU; I had always felt a strong desire to breast-feed him.

"Hello, my name is Ali Barton, and I just gave birth to a thirty-one-weeker who is in the NICU.

I would like the lactation consultant to bring me a breast pump and show me how to use it."

"She is out on the floor right now, what room are you in?" the receptionist asked.

"I am actually in the ICU, not in labor and delivery."

She took a sharp breath, and took my name and room number. One hour later, I still had no pump. I called three more times, and hours later, a lactation consultant from the NICU came to show me how to operate the pump. She set me up, and to my delight, I was able to pump a few drops of colostrum for Andrew to bring back to Ethan.

Andrew came back from the NICU to check on me. My parents and Emily had arrived and had seen Ethan in his incubator. They all came in to tell me how beautiful he was, and how well he was doing.

"They put him on something called a CPAP, which helps him a little with his breathing, but they did not need to intubate him," Andrew said, his face lit up with delight. "He is doing so great, hon. I'm so proud of you!"

"That's great! I'm so happy," I said. My eyes welled up with tears. I was frustrated that I could not hold my son in my arms. I was stuck in this bed, and all I wanted to do was be in the NICU.

Andrew came to my side and wrapped his arms around me. "You'll be out of here before you know it, and then we can go see him together."

I nodded and handed him a tube of milk. "Bring this to him. He must be hungry." Andrew left with my sister to go back to the NICU.

The rest of the time in the ICU was a blur. I felt manic with excitement that we had both lived through the birth, defying the expectations of all the doctors. Ethan was small but thriving, and in those moments, I knew everything would be okay.

Dr. Economy came to check on me as she had so many nights in the hospital in Shapiro. "He is beautiful, Ali." She had been to the NICU to visit him. "You did it. I am so proud of you." She squeezed my hand. "Doctors don't like to be proven wrong, but in this case I am really happy that you proved us all wrong."

The doctors wanted me to stay in bed because of the risk of fluid shifts leading to heart failure post birth, but I felt amazing. I knew I was going to be fine. In those moments, I felt I would never need a heart transplant. I knew they were all wrong.

I can't recall what I did to pass the time before I got to go see Ethan. I was restless, yet I was not allowed to get out of bed. Doctors came to check on me, nurses checked my vital signs every hour, and I passed the time by gazing at the photos that my parents had taken in the NICU.

Emily came back to my room. "Wait until you see this, Ali. This is amazing," she said, coming to my bedside. She handed me her phone with a video ready to play. I will never forget that video and still tear up to this day when I think about it. Ethan was crying, his cries sounding like a little kitten, not developed enough yet to have a real baby cry. I watched as Andrew took a small cotton swab, and as instructed by the NICU nurse, dipped the swab into my tube of colostrum and wiped it in Ethan's mouth.

Emily explained, "They told us his tummy is so little now, all he needs is a very little bit. You are feeding him! They said if you can pump more milk he won't need any formula!"

I began to sob. I was so happy to see Ethan calm down when he had my milk. I was overwhelmed by the intensity of my emotions while watching the video.

Emily rubbed my back. "You will see him soon, Ali. You will hold him real soon."

In that moment, I made it my mission to pump every two hours for twenty minutes, exactly as the lactation consultant had instructed. If I couldn't hold my baby and nurture him in my arms, I would give him milk and nurture him from the ICU as best as I could.

The next day, I was discharged from my bed. The nurses wanted to check my blood pressure while sitting, standing, and then after walking. I did what was instructed, huffing and glaring with impatience. After completing what seemed like endless paperwork, I was discharged out of the ICU and back into Shapiro.

Chapter 17

My Baby

MY NURSE TOOK ME TO THE NICU IN A WHEEL-chair with Andrew by my side. I could barely sit still in the chair, eager to hold Ethan. From around the corner, I saw a brown blanket with farm animals that my sister had made for Ethan draped over the top of an incubator.

"They try to mimic the womb as much as they can, so they keep it dark in there," Andrew explained to me. The nurses had us wash our hands and use hand sanitizer, before rolling me over to a reclining chair. I lifted the edge of the blanket to see Ethan's eyes open and looking around.

"Do you want to hold him?" the nurse asked.

Andrew laughed. "I think she has been waiting her whole life to hold him."

I leaned back in the chair and the nurse handed me a warm blanket. "Why don't you take your shirt off, so you can do skin to skin? It is really good for the baby to get that contact."

As I took off my shirt, she took Ethan out, slow and cautious. There were thick tubes around his face, helping him to breathe. He also had a small orange tube going into his nose, feeding him my pumped milk at timed intervals. He was crying, that small kitten noise, and my eyes welled up with tears again. The moment she placed him on my chest, he stopped crying.

"Hi, my sweet Ethan," I said, sobbing. "I love you so much." I looked up at Andrew. "I love you," I mouthed to him. We sat in silence, gazing at Ethan and taking pictures of him. Lying on my chest, his tiny feet rested above my belly button, flopping out on my belly. I couldn't believe they were my baby's feet. After a few minutes, he fell fast asleep on my chest. An hour before, I had been given my dose of diuretics. I had to use the bathroom, but there was no way I was moving from that chair.

"I would do this all over again in a heartbeat to have this moment. This makes it all worth it," I said to Andrew. He squeezed my hand, and he nodded. We both knew I had made the right decision.

We sat there for hours, and I sang, "You Are My Sunshine," as I had done to my belly throughout the pregnancy.

The doctors decided to keep me in the hospital for a few weeks to keep me monitored. For once, I was not eager to be at home in my own bed. I wanted to be within five minutes of Ethan and didn't want to go home until could come with me.

My nurses were sweet enough to bring me to the NICU whenever I wanted, even sometimes in the middle of the night if I could not sleep. I pumped around the clock, making sure to set my alarm for every two hours to get my milk over to Ethan. The doctors had told me they did not think I would be able to breastfeed. I was still on high doses of diuretics, and they thought that this would affect my supply. I was told it was safe to breastfeed, but they did not think my supply would last.

I was determined to prove them wrong again and impressed the NICU nurses with the multiple bottles I brought to them every few hours. They directed me to send some home with Andrew to start saving in the freezer.

I became obsessed with my daily beverages. It was torture to be a breastfeeding mother on diuretics with a set limit of one and a half liters of fluid a day. I planned my day according to the drinks people would bring me.

I told my mom, "I had my cup of tea this morning, but if you bring me an iced decaf from Starbucks, that can last me through tonight and I can still have two bottles of water."

I constantly paced the hallways and sucked on ice. My mouth was dry, and all I could think about was sneaking more water, which I often did. The nurses would come in multiple times a day to ask for my fluid intake, and the cafeteria was instructed to limit the amount of fluid they could serve to me. A bucket was placed in my bathroom to measure my urine output, and my dose of IV diuretic was administered accordingly.

When Ethan was three weeks old, I got a call from the hospital's public relations department, eager to do a story on us. We arranged for them to meet us in the NICU to do a video interview. Today, I can sit back and watch this interview and I am astounded by my level of denial.

"So according to your doctors, it sounds like you are going to be listed for a heart transplant. Do you have a lot of family and friends supporting you?"

I interrupted the interviewer before she could continue. "I am feeling great now that Ethan is here. Maybe eventually one day I will need one. Medical technology is so amazing now. By then there will be some alternative to transplant that is much less invasive. I just want to go home with my son and live a normal life with my family."

Chapter 18

The NICU

AFTER TWO WEEKS OF BEING STABLE, THE DOC-
tors decided to discharge me and then follow
me daily on an outpatient basis. I was spending all
day, seven days a week at the NICU. Ethan and I sat
in our little corner, where I sang to him, nursed him,
bathed and changed him, and took thousands of
photos and videos of him. The nurses had decorated
his area with photos and drawings, and I brought
in preemie clothing and other decorations to make
it feel like home. There was no privacy, except for
screens we could use when I nursed. After a few
days, I was able to block out all the beeps from the
machines, even the scary sounding ones. It was just
me and Ethan in there.

Initially, everything seemed to go wrong. He had
a small brain hemorrhage, a hole in his heart, and he
would stop breathing when he nursed or took a bottle of my milk. I will never forget the terrible sound
of his monitor going off when he would stop breathing. As a nurse rushed over, I would gently tap his
chest area, trying to arouse him, or kiss the top of

his head. All these problems self-resolved by thirty-five weeks, and my tiny little wrinkly creature was turning into a little baby. I felt guilty when I left him at the end of the day to sleep at home but knew he was well cared for, and I would be back the next day. His nurses Felicia and Kristine loved and cared for Ethan as if he was their own.

In the meantime, the doctors wanted to set me up for a full heart catheterization, echocardiogram, and exercise stress test to see how the heart looked post birth. If my fluid retention and exhaustion were any indication, things were not good. Every few days, I would wake up and have gained ten pounds. The doctors would have me come to clinic and get on an IV infusion of diuretics for four hours, after which I would lose all the weight, rush to pump in the NICU, and then hold Ethan until I left to go home that night.

I kept pushing off the testing, since I knew the results would not be good. I was not yet ready to face the reality of my condition.

Chapter 19

Ethan Comes Home

Ethan finally came home after seven long weeks in the NICU. It was March 20, 2014, and we were ecstatic. It felt bizarre to snuggle with him on our couch. No wires, tubes, or beeping. We were home as a family. Ethan slept in a bassinet by my bedside, and life was getting back to our norm.

In April, the team scheduled me for my testing. The results were worse than expected. They could not believe that I was able to walk around and care for Ethan alone. A third of my heart was pumping properly, while the other two-thirds was stiffening and losing elasticity. It was getting worse as the days passed. My kidneys and liver were poorly functioning.

Suddenly, we were scheduling an appointment to have a family meeting with my cardiologist, Dr. Lakdawala, to make some decisions.

My mom, dad, Andrew and I sat squeezed in a small exam room. I sat on the table, nursing Ethan with a cover over me. Dr. Lakdawala locked eyes with me. "Ali, a transplant is not an easy fix. When you get a transplant, you trade one problem for different problems. We want to delay getting this until we feel it is absolutely necessary. Once you get a transplant, it is almost like a ticking time bomb. They don't last forever, and given that you are so young, you would be looking at eventually needing another one."

I looked down at Ethan, angry that I was sitting in that office, hearing what felt like a death sentence.

He continued, "The medications cause their own host of issues. The anti-rejection medications are something you will need to take for the rest of your entire life. Your immune system will always be suppressed, and you will have to be very careful about getting infections. It also will make you more likely to get cancer and other diseases."

Tears formed in my eyes, and Andrew rubbed my back.

"I'm sorry, Ali. I know this is a lot of information, but I am just trying to tell you the reality of the situation. A transplant is not a fix. I do think that if you have the means, you should travel outside of New England. The wait here is long, and sometimes you have to get really sick and live in the hospital before you may or may not get an organ in time. I know your dad has done some research on possibly going to Tampa General Hospital. If we want to look into that more, we are happy to talk to the team there and set up an evaluation."

My dad nodded as I wiped my tears off the top of Ethan's head.

I left the office depressed and exhausted. All I could think about was leaving Ethan and Andrew. I felt defeated and extremely sorry for myself.

Andrew tried to rub my shoulder as we walked, my parents trailing behind us. "It's going to be ok, hon," he said.

Tears welled up in my eyes, and I sped up. I started to get out of breath as he caught up with me. Per usual, I tried to hide my breathlessness and not say anything to Andrew. I could not hide anything. He knew how sick I was, and how I was declining. He was in a constant panic over me staying home alone all day with Ethan. I argued with everyone, saying I was fine and I could do it alone. I had been robbed of my ability to enjoy the first few months of Ethan's life. Instead, the thought was buzzing in my head that I could die any second, and that I may not make it to the surgery even if I had a transplant.

My days were scheduled around taking my maximum dose of prescribed diuretics twice a day at 8 a.m. and 3 p.m., then lying flat for one hour afterward. The lying flat was to ensure that the medication sent the signal to my kidneys to allow me to urinate and get rid of the excess fluid my body loved to hold on to because of my heart's failure to pump properly. I wondered how I could manage that when Ethan became mobile.

I walked with Ethan in his stroller in between feedings and medication time, insisting I was fine to walk and that I needed some normalcy in my routine. Seeing a "normal" mom made me feel sorry for myself, an attitude not beneficial for my mind or my body.

After the meeting, I glanced down at Ethan, calm and asleep in his stroller. "I don't get it," I said to Andrew. I caught my breath as I noticed a young mom walking by us in the opposite direction, pushing her stroller in front of her with no apparent effort.

"I don't get what? Maybe we should try to call Tampa later?" Andrew's voice wavered. He was trying to stay strong for me.

"This isn't what life should be like," I said, raising my voice, tears flowing freely. "I have always tried so hard to be healthy and fit, I always take good care of myself. I just don't get why I am here. I should be enjoying Ethan and now I have to move to Florida? What the fuck? I can't deal with this anymore."

He grabbed my hand and stopped me from walking. People stared at us. "You have to stay positive. We are going to get through this together." He wrapped his arms around me, and Ethan started to stir.

"Let's keep walking so he won't wake up," I said, moving forward. This was my habit, to push people away when my emotions became too intense. I felt regret for dragging so many others into my mess.

Andrew was anxious and overwhelmed, and I felt I had destroyed his life and his sanity when he married me. I was broken, and all I did was bring him anxiety, nothing else. Between that, the IVF, and now this impending transplant, I felt as if I would be better alone, so that I would not drag everyone down with me.

We all loaded into the car once we got to the medical garage. The ride was silent; my family knew me well enough to know I did not want to talk about this.

When we got to the house, I unlatched Ethan's car seat, and said, "I'll call Tampa tomorrow." I had to get over this attitude. Feeling sorry for myself or jealous of "normal" moms was not going to make me healthy.

Andrew took Ethan's car seat out of my hands and kissed me. "I think that is a really good decision."

Chapter 20

Planning

THE NEXT DAY, I CALLED MY CONTACT, TAMMI Wicks at Tampa General. She had already been in communication with one of my Brigham nurses. After asking me a few questions, Tammi was ready to schedule my evaluation. She was friendly and helpful, and I immediately felt comfortable with her as my primary nurse coordinator. I was officially on the transplant list in Boston, and any time I accumulated would transfer down to Florida.

It was April, and we decided that I would come down for Memorial Day Weekend for two days of testing. I felt sad that I would miss the family tradition of spending the long weekend in Rhode Island, but I knew it was important to get moving with our plans. Tammi explained to me that after the evaluation, I could choose when I wanted to move down to Tampa. The testing was a formality, and she assured me that since I was listed in Boston, it should not be an issue to be accepted on the Tampa list.

"I also think it should be a pretty short wait. Since you are smaller than our average transplant patient, you can't get a large heart, just like a large person can't get a small heart," Tammi said. "There are very few people of your size and weight on the list. I can't give you an exact time, but I have seen some patients get the call two weeks after arriving. More conservatively I would say between three to six months. We are also going to try giving you an IV of a medication called milrinone, that should help the functioning of your heart. It will also move you up to 1B status and increase the chances of a faster transplant."

In Boston, I was status two, meaning I was living at home and functioning. In New England, this means you most likely will never get a call for a transplant, until you get sick enough to move to 1A (living in the hospital and near death) or 1B (living at home, with some sort of home intervention such as an IV or a ventricular assist device). Brigham did not want to do milrinone with me, since they felt there were more risks of abnormal rhythm. I would need to wear a life vest to shock me in case of emergency.

Tammi continued, "Also, we will keep an eye on your liver and kidney functioning. If it looks like either is worsening, we will hospitalize you and you would move to 1A status."

My liver and kidneys had been severely affected by the heart failure. This was being monitored several times a week by the team.

After I finished the call, I checked to make sure Ethan was still napping in his bassinet. I texted

Andrew to check on the dates and then booked our flights to Tampa. Then, I wrote a message to the family, trying to be lighthearted: "Tampa, here we come!" I was petrified, but wanted to get this done and move on with my life.

I was exhausted yet energized by Ethan, who had developed a little personality by four months old. Nothing made me happier than spending the day with him. He provided me with distraction in the best possible way from all my medical problems. Since I felt so tired from the heart failure, much of my day was spent with visitors and snuggling with Ethan. We had finally got into a pattern with his sleep, but I was still pumping every two to three hours on top of nursing for about forty-five minutes per session. I was "on" all the time and running myself ragged.

Ethan would sleep in small chunks during the day, and every night he would wake at midnight, three and six. I became fixated on obtaining enough breast milk to get him through his first birthday, and this meant obsessively pumping and storing my milk in our deep freezer. In addition, I had several wonderful friends who had offered to pump extra. I had a large reserve in our freezer ready to go for after my transplant. I had major anxiety about Ethan developing normally because of his prematurity. We went to the pediatrician weekly for weight checks. The contrast between my doctors panicking over a three pound weight gain in one day for me, and Ethan's pediatrician panicking about his weight gain of less than half to one ounce per day was almost laughable.

In retrospect, obsessing and focusing on Ethan's development and nutrition was a way for me to redirect my nervous energy about my impending surgery. I have always been a control freak with a tinge of an obsessive compulsive personality disorder, so I controlled what I could, which was ensuring that my baby boy grew up healthy and strong. Ethan was seen weekly for Early Intervention, and I felt moments of guilt knowing that I would be taking him away from his therapists while we went to Florida.

Chapter 21

Tampa General Hospital

THE EVALUATION WEEKEND FINALLY CAME. WE were staying in small accommodations for patients next door to the hospital, and arrived the evening before my evaluation. I had no idea what I would be asked to do at these tests. I had been told on the phone, but at this point I felt that my brain was not retaining any information. I was tired and getting sicker by the day. My lips were constantly purple, and my body seemed to be deteriorating.

We arrived at our room and quickly realized that there were no restaurants nearby. "Hospital cafeteria it is!" I joked. We crossed the street to Tampa General, finding the cafeteria closed. We found a bar and restaurant by searching on our phones, but it was one mile down the road.

Andrew looked at me with concern. "Why don't I walk down and bring us back some stuff," he said.

I felt nervous to be alone with Ethan in a strange place. "Hon, I'll be fine. I can walk there! No big deal!"

With Ethan snoozing in his stroller, we began

to move towards the restaurant at a slow pace. It was unpleasantly humid and hot outside, and I felt myself trying to catch a deep breath. Andrew could tell I was struggling and offered to push the stroller.

When we finally sat down to eat what felt like hours later, I was no longer in denial. I needed a transplant, and I wanted it as soon as possible. I hated the fact that Andrew had to ask for an extra chair for me so that I could elevate my legs at the table. I hated that I was so tired and uncomfortable and swollen that I could not enjoy dinner with my husband and son. Most of all, I hated what my life had turned into, and how limited I was. I hated that I needed to even be in Tampa. I should have been enjoying my family weekend in Rhode Island.

The next day we arrived at the hospital. The nurses told me that Ethan would have to be apart from me, and I lost my cool. This was not off to a good start. "I'm not doing the testing then," I insisted like a child. "He is breastfeeding, and I can't leave him."

They finally agreed to allow him in. Andrew would temporarily take him when I was rolled in for various tests such as a catheritization and X-ray. I had met my doctor, Dr. Mackie, and my nurse coordinator Tammi and instantly felt comfortable in their care. They made me feel at home, taking the time to get to know me.

"How long will I have to go without seeing Ethan after my surgery?" I asked.

Tammi put her hand on my shoulder and said, "I know how hard this is. I have kids too. Ethan won't be able to come to the ICU after transplant, but we will definitely find a way to sneak him in when you are on a cardiac recovery floor. Most people are in the hospital anywhere from ten days to a few weeks, depending on their recovery. Since you are young and otherwise healthy, I think you will be home before you know it!"

After transplant education, including long discussions with Dr. Mackie about the transplant process, I thought the day was finished.

Then a nurse told me, "We are going to start you on something called milrinone. This is not safe for breastfeeding, so you will not be able to feed Ethan after we start the IV. We will be keeping you overnight to monitor you. This should help you feel a lot better."

"What?" I shouted. "I didn't bring enough milk for him, and no one told me I would have to sleep here! No!" The nurse looked shocked. I looked down at Ethan in my arms and back up at Andrew. "No," I repeated.

A few conversations later, and after a lot of Google research, we found a more nursing-friendly IV medication called dobutamine, which they told me I would be taking once I arrived to Tampa. Being on an IV at home would move me up on the list, and this medication was supposed to make my heart beat more efficiently. They agreed to try it for a few hours, and then let me sleep at the hotel that night if all went well.

Ethan was getting fussier as the day went on. He was hungry, tired, and therefore crying hysterically. Nothing I did made him stop. I pulled everything out of my bag of tricks: songs, humming, tickling, swaying, shooshing, swaddling. He was hysterical and would not latch onto my breast. I finally asked for a pump from the NICU, and Ethan took a bottle once I had pumped the milk.

I looked up at Andrew when Ethan finally calmed down. He held my hand. "This is the worst day ever. I just want to go home." He nodded, and I saw his eyes well up with tears also.

Shortly after arriving back home in Boston, we found out that Tampa accepted me as a patient. Tammi called to tell me the good news. "Now you just need to decide when you want to come."

"I think I already sorted out our housing," I said. "My dad found a furnished apartment in Tampa that does month-to-month rentals. How long do you think I will need to stay after the surgery?"

"That's great that you found housing! I think if you come down within the month, you are going to be right up there on the list. Things should move quickly. Dr. Mackie said if everything goes smoothly and you are recovering well, we could send you back a month after your discharge from the hospital."

"Awesome!" In my head, I was prepared to be back to Boston for Labor Day Weekend, where

I could enjoy the end of the summer at home. It almost seemed too easy. "Let me call the rental agent and discuss it with my family, and I can get back to you later."

Tammi agreed, and I hung up to call Andrew and work, then my parents and siblings. An hour later, I called her back. "We will come out on June 20th." I swallowed a lump. June 20th was in three weeks.

My dad always used to call me a right-now-nick. When I made my mind up about something, I would make it happen as soon as I could. I just wanted this transplant to be done with. The faster I got to Tampa, the faster I would start my life as a mom the way I saw it should be. I was packed and ready to go two weeks before we left. Every day I lived with endomyocardial fibrosis was a day taken away from Andrew and Ethan. I wanted to be a mom who was there for my son, take him to activities, and be present. I couldn't do that while I was sick. I could only think about how much I hated this illness. I hated that it was taking the spark out of my life.

Chapter 22

Saying Goodbye

IN THE WEEKS LEADING UP TO OUR DEPARTURE, WE made all the logistical plans: shipping my car down, deciding who would take turns coming down to stay with me and Ethan while Andrew worked, finding Ethan a pediatrician, packing our belongings. Before I knew it, I was saying my goodbyes with my closest friends.

My last afternoon in Boston was eighty degrees and beautiful. I was leaving it for the oppressive June heat in Florida, and I regretted having to say goodbye to my best friends that afternoon. I remember the day so well. I could tell Alexis, Tracy, and Emily were furious that I had walked a mile in the heat to have our final goodbye at Panera the day before I left. No one wanted to say it. No one wanted to fight before I left. Everyone walked on eggshells around me. If anyone confronted me on my health choices or decisions about my physical activities, I would get defensive and angry. Everyone wanted to keep the peace. In my eyes, I had been through so much, and I was angry at the world. I wanted my sense of normal and control, and I wanted to pretend I was like any other healthy mom who could casually walk over the coffee shop to meet her girlfriends. The reality was, I could not be that cool, casual, and spontaneous mom. I was too sick.

I shouldn't have been walking around with Ethan in the heat; no one could predict how long it would be before my heart just gave out. Everyone else knew that—it was clear as day—but I was in denial. I still wasn't even 100% sure transplant was the answer, although I was more than ready to leave this sad existence behind and find out.

Chapter 23

Our New Home

AFTER A LONG BUT SUCCESSFUL FLIGHT WHERE Ethan nursed and slept the entire trip, I opened the door to our apartment in Tampa, and breathed a sigh of relief.

"It's nice!" I yelled back to Andrew, who was rolling our luggage down the hallway. The apartment was nicely furnished and clean. When Andrew entered, I had already laid Ethan down on a mat to change his diaper.

"Wow! This is great," Andrew said. "Let's go check things out!"

It was late afternoon, ninety degrees and humid. Ethan was alert and awake. I picked him up and we walked slowly down the hallway towards the pool area, Andrew's hand on my lower back as if I could collapse at any time.

"Do you think he's hungry again? Maybe we should try a bottle this time so he can get used to it." Tears welled up in my eyes. The team at home and in Tampa felt very strongly that I should be weaning Ethan from breastfeeding. Tammi had emphasized that I could get a call very quickly, and if Ethan were not at least partially weaned, it would be a lot harder for both of us.

I had promised the team I would start the process, but I had not. I was holding on to the last physical thing I could provide for Ethan. I felt too sad and emotional about taking away that bond we had. I was ready to try one bottle of pumped milk each day with him for practice, but I wanted to nurse him until the very last moment. We had purchased a deep freezer for Florida, and my parents planned to ship me my frozen milk via our Fed Ex account.

I had also met some wonderful moms through my mommy groups who promised extra pumping sessions to provide milk for Ethan. My friend Amanda had filled our deep freezer at home before we had left; another friend, Emily, had over two thousand ounces to send us while we were there. Andrew planned to pick up milk from my friends Bridget and Kristina when he went back to Boston. Several other moms had also rallied to bring milk to Andrew. I felt utterly loved and grateful that I had amazing friends who cared enough to do this for Ethan.

"Look!" Andrew said, interrupting my thought process. I looked straight ahead at a beautiful empty swimming pool surrounded by palm trees and beach chairs. I smiled, feeling conflicted because on one hand I felt like this was a vacation; and on the other hand, I just wanted to be back at home in Boston, not having to endure this medical stuff.

He came up behind me and rubbed my shoulders. "This is going to fly by, hon. Before you know it, you'll get the call and you'll be back at home by the end of the summer!"

I closed my eyes and leaned back into his arms. "I hate this," I whispered. "How am I going to do this without you here?" I wiped away a tear that had fallen into Ethan's hair.

"Your mom and dad will be here Sunday night, and we are going to try to have someone with you as much as we can. And if no one else can be here, your parents want you to have a nurse."

I rolled my eyes. "No," I said, walking away. "I'm not having a stranger stay with me. I'm fine! I can take care of Ethan alone. Everyone needs to just calm down. Angela will start in few weeks, and I am totally fine overnight."

I had found Angela a few weeks earlier on care. com. Se was planning on helping care for Ethan after my surgery since I would not be able to lift him or care for him alone. We planned on introducing her before the surgery, to allow Ethan to get used to and become comfortable with her.

"Ali, we already talked about this. You don't know what could happen! And how would you feel if something did happen to you and no one was here to watch Ethan or call 911 for you?"

I rolled my eyes again and argued, "I have gotten through the past four years with undiagnosed heart failure. I have taught my classes, run, walked, and birthed a baby. All of it has been fine. I'm still not even 100 percent convinced that I should be here! Everyone needs to calm down. It's going to be fine." Andrew gave a deep sigh.

We had had the same conversation over and over. I didn't want any help. I could do it all alone. When I was caring for Ethan, I never thought about all of this heart transplant drama. I was infatuated with motherhood, and he kept me going. I knew Ethan would get me through this anxious waiting period.

Leading up to this time, I had connected with several other transplant patients. I learned from them that the time you wait for the transplant is the worst; every time your phone rings, it could be "the call." I was anxious enough already, and nervously anticipated this wait. At home, Ethan and I had a routine going with play dates and activities. I was nervous about having so much empty time. Too much open time would lead to me getting too much in my own head, leading to resentment and feeling sorry for myself, and then obsessing about feeling out of control in my body. I just wanted distractions at this point.

"We'll talk about it later," Andrew responded. "Do you want me to hold Ethan, and we can go back inside and unpack?"

"I can hold him." I always held him. I didn't want to let go. I was scared of what was going to happen once I did let go. I wanted to hold him as much as possible in case anything happened during the transplant. Just as it began to drizzle, we headed back inside.

Two days later, it was time for Andrew to go back home to Boston and return to work. I was in a sour mood all day, although looking forward to my parents arriving to take over for him. The family planned on switching off staying with us; my sister was coming the following week.

My car had been delivered, full of toys, more clothes, and all the baby stuff. I dropped Andrew off at the airport. He was coming back in two weekends, but it felt like forever.

"I love you so much, bubs. It's going to be fine," he said as he brushed the tears away from my eyes. I had cried more in that last week than I ever had. I was sick of crying. I tried to mentally force myself to toughen up and stop.

"Love you, too. I'll see you before you know it. I'll face time you tonight," I said, looking away. Ethan was fast asleep in his car seat.

"I hope Ethan doesn't forget me! Make sure you call me when he's awake. Or if you need me to talk to him tonight when he won't go to sleep." We laughed, and Andrew squeezed my hand.

The first few nights in Tampa, Ethan had turned into a night owl, with his witching hour starting at six until about nine. He would cry and refuse sleep; no matter what we did, he would be miserable and hysterical. The only thing that seemed to soothe him was the sound of the vacuum cleaner, which we ran almost constantly in the corner of the room during those hours.

"You're so strong, hon. You can do this." Andrew gave us both kisses, and then took his bags out of the trunk and left, waving as he entered the doors to the airport.

I looked in the review mirror at Ethan, peaceful in his sleep. And then I panicked. I was alone. In Florida, I didn't know anyone, I didn't know what to do with myself. So I decided to drive Ethan to the Whole Foods in Tampa to get a coffee and sit down and read until my parent's flight arrived that evening.

My mom and dad knocked on the door right after I had finally gotten Ethan to settle for the evening. I wrapped myself in their arms, so happy to have people to talk to again that day.

"How are you feeling?" my dad asked as he placed his luggage in their bedroom.

"I feel ok! I'm ready for this appointment tomorrow to see where things stand with the list, and how they think I am doing. Not looking forward to having the IV placed."

My dad nodded. "It shouldn't hurt. I'm pretty sure they will put you under. It should be interesting to see if the dobutamine helps you to feel better."

I tilted my head towards my bedroom, hearing a noise from Ethan. I peeked in the room and saw him squirming around in the pack and play. My parents and I chatted for a few minutes, then I decided to go lay down in preparation for being at the hospital early in the morning. The doctors would place a PICC line in my chest area to run the medication into my heart. This IV would allow me to move up to 1B status on the list and was supposed to help my heart function slightly better until the transplant.

The next morning Dr. Mackie and Tammi walked into the exam room with warm smiles on their faces. I immediately felt at home with them, as they cooed at Ethan and welcomed us to Tampa. Dr. Mackie explained the process of the PICC placement, and we talked about the waiting period.

"Ali, we are going to monitor you every few days. As you know, your kidneys and your liver are affected by the heart failure. We are going to get labs every few days, and if they show further signs of decline, we would hospitalize you and move you to 1A status. You would get the heart even faster that way."

I nodded, nervously glancing towards my parents. I wanted to wait at home and not be away from Ethan for any longer than I needed to be. "The IV dobutamine will help," Dr. Mackie continued. "A nurse is going to come to your apartment later today to show you how to properly change the medication bag. You will need to have a backup battery pack and machine with you at all times. The medication will be delivered to you as needed. You keep it in the fridge. Also, a nurse will come by every few days to change the dressing on the PICC line. When you are on the infusion, you are supposed to wear a life vest that could shock you in case of emergency."

"A life vest? Seriously? Isn't that overkill? I thought I wasn't at risk for abnormal rhythms with it since that is not the norm for my condition." Ethan began to cry, and I took out my nursing cover to feed him.

Tammi gently patted me on my back. "How is the weaning going? Ali, it's really important that you get Ethan used to a bottle." I nodded again, not answering her question.

"I don't think you are at risk for abnormal rhythms with the IV. It is just a precaution," Dr. Mackie said. "A representative from the life vest company will come show you how to use it."

I looked at my parents, sitting in the corner looking stressed and anxious. "So if I wear the life vest, what happens if I am shocked while I am holding Ethan?" I asked, nervous about my answer.

"That's a good question. You would get a warning alarm to indicate you were about to be shocked, so I would suggest putting Ethan on the ground. However, if you lost consciousness, this would be something to be worried about. This is why we suggest having someone around you at all times. That is one of the reasons your parents want to get you a nurse for when they are not there."

In that moment, I made the decision I would not wear that vest. It felt like it was 100 degrees that day, and the thought of wearing a bulky vest that could perhaps kill Ethan by accidentally shocking him convinced me to leave the vest in my closet when it arrived. I had read all the articles on dobutamine, and the chances were very slim for me to develop an abnormal rhythm.

"We will discuss the nurse thing again with Ali later," my mom said.

"No, we won't," I said under my breath. I knew I was acting like a child, but I felt so scared and frustrated with the entire situation. I was exhausted from lack of sleep. Ethan was waking every ninety minutes to nurse during the night, and the anticipatory anxiety left me unable to shut my eyes. It was almost as if Ethan knew something different and scary was coming, and he was regressing back to his newborn sleep schedule.

"Ali, it's not something to take lightly. Only one third of your heart is functioning right now, and even that one third isn't doing a whole lot. I know you think you feel okay, but it is better to be safe than sorry," Dr. Mackie said. "You are right at the top of the list in your weight category. Being so small is definitely helpful in this situation. Since you are doing all right, we are going to wait until the best possible heart comes for you. We won't take just anything. In the meantime, keep taking the maximum dose of the torsemide diuretic during the day, twice a day. That should keep the fluid off."

As he was talking, a stretcher came in for me. I handed Ethan off to my dad and waved goodbye as they rolled me down the hallway.

Chapter 24

Waiting

DAYS LATER, I WENT IN FOR A FOLLOW UP WITH Dr. Mackie to see how I was adjusting to the dobutamine. As he had me lean back and turn my head to the left to check my jugular, he told me he had an offer for a heart, but the team had decided to pass.

"What, already? That was so fast! What happened?" I asked. In that moment, everything became real, and I realized I was not yet emotionally prepared to get the call.

"It was a sixty-year-old woman with a history of drug abuse, not ideal for you. Like I said before, we don't want to take just any heart for you, unless it is an emergency. Your liver enzymes and kidney function have actually improved since you started the dobutamine, so we want to wait for the perfect heart." I nodded my head in agreement, relieved but also disappointed that the heart wasn't the right one for me.

He sat down on a stool next to me. "Have you been keeping busy with Ethan? How are you guys liking it here? I have a bunch of places I'll write down for you to visit; good restaurants, farmers' markets, beaches. Something to help pass the time, right?"

I laughed. "I feel like I am about to have a heart attack every time my phone rings, Dr. Mackie. I need good distractions! To be honest, Ethan has been sleeping so poorly that I wouldn't mind a good night's sleep with some anesthesia."

He smiled and chuckled. "Just wait, they only get worse. I'll show you a video of my toddler climbing out of her pack and play." He showed me a cute video on his phone as I giggled. In that moment, I knew I would be fine. Dr. Mackie was genuinely caring, and he would do his best to make sure I got the best heart possible.

My parents were set to leave the next day. I had a gap of four days before my sister came. My parents insisted on a night visiting nurse and begged me to call to set it up. I knew Andrew was worried and this would help him feel better, although I dreaded it.

The first night was the worse. A large Jamaican woman walked into my house and made me feel like I was completely disabled and incapable of doing anything. When Ethan cried, she swooped into his room and lifted him out of the crib to start rocking him.

"Um, excuse me, I can do that. I think he wants to nurse," I said timidly. She shushed me and walked into the guest room with Ethan.

I called Andrew. "I'm not doing this!" I whispered to him, furious.

"Ali, just go in there and take Ethan," he said.

"I can't," I insisted. "She took him away and didn't listen to me. He's hungry and it's time for him to eat!"

"Go in there and take him. And tomorrow we'll call the company and explain that you don't need that kind of help."

I hung up the phone with him, walked into the guest room and reached my arms out, trying to hold back my tears and anger. "Please hand me my son. It's time for him to eat and I can do this."

She looked up at me. "I'm sorry. I am just doing my job."

"It's not your job to take my son from me. It's your job to make sure I don't die in the middle of the night." With that, I walked away holding Ethan, and then shut the door to my room.

The next day, Andrew told me a new nurse would be coming the following night. "This is so stupid." I said, frustrated with strangers in my home.

"I know you think it's stupid, but I'm afraid something is going to happen to you while you're with Ethan. Please just do this for me."

I agreed and endured two more nights of sitting awkwardly on the couch while some woman sat next to me watching my every move and following me around the house like I could break at any minute.

Finally, the night before my sister was scheduled to arrive, the nurse did not show at 9 p.m. as she was supposed to. I had my first peaceful night since my parents had left. I told no one.

My sister arrived the next day. We made plans to visit the farmers market, go swimming, and take a trip to the Hyde Park area. I had been in Tampa for only two weeks, but it felt like forever.

I was so happy to see my sister again. The first evening, we waded in the pool as Ethan napped in the stroller next to us. I had developed a way to get in the pool with my IV by holding the medication bag on my shoulder like a boom box from the 1990s.

I told my sister my frustration about the night nurses and wanting to get back to my old life before I got sick.

She said, "Ali, we are all worried about you. You have to cut the shit and just let people help you. You are in complete denial about how sick you are, and everyone is just scared shitless. Put yourself in our shoes."

My eyes filled up. Everyone walked on eggshells with me, but Emily always called me on my stupid behavior choices. "Put yourself in my shoes, pook. This sucks. I can't do anything I want. No one understands how this feels. No one."

"I know, Ali. This is temporary. I know you would never forgive yourself if something happened to

Ethan because you insisted on being alone with him all the time. Like these long walks you take with him in the morning. What if you collapsed? Or driving around Tampa? Seriously, Ali. You love Ethan more than anything and you're such an amazing mom, but you are in so much denial. None of us want to see anything bad happen."

I got up and walked away, taking Ethan with me. I was furious and needed some space. I took a walk around the apartment area. After thirty minutes, I realized that I was angry because she was absolutely right. I was trying to maintain my sense of normalcy, when there was nothing about the situation that was normal. I was sick and could die at any moment. And here I was with my baby, walking in the heat and taking him to the coffee shop so I could sit and read and pretend that my life as I knew it had not been completely flipped upside down.

I called Emily's cell. "You're right, pook. I'm coming back. I just needed some space to think. I got so mad because everything you said is true."

A few more days passed, and Emily went home. I spent three more nights with my nurses before Andrew would come, followed by my dad a few days later.

When Andrew arrived, I sobbed as I threw himself into his arms. We spent the weekend snuggling with Ethan and taking day trips for sightseeing.

Andrew was cautious of how far we walked and always checked to make sure I wasn't overdoing it. We made trips to Whole Foods often. It felt like home to me since it had been a common meet-up place with friends in Boston.

"I'm sick of waiting. I want this to be over with," I told him, as we sat enjoying iced coffee on the patio at our favorite coffee shop. Ethan looked up at me, and I kissed the top of his head. I shifted in my seat. I felt sweat accumulate from where Ethan was lying on my chest in the baby carrier.

"I bet it will happen any day," Andrew said, hugging me and kissing my cheek. "I bet when I go home I'll get a call telling me to turn around and come back."

Tammi had been in contact after my labs came in, telling me they had two more offers of hearts that they didn't think would be a good match.

"I know it's bad, but I just want them to accept the next one!" I swiveled the sugar in the bottom of my coffee with my straw. My patience was dwindling.

"It will be soon."

My dad arrived the next day after Andrew left, and we kept busy visiting local stores and strolling around town. That evening, my dad told me that Mom had wanted to come too, but wasn't feeling well enough. "The wait" was stressing her out and exacerbating her medical condition. My mom suffers with dopa responsive dystonia and has symptoms similar to Parkinson's disease. She gets rigid and stiff when she gets stressed. Dad thought it would be better if she stayed at home this time.

Dad and I ate a home-cooked grilled fish and salad dinner together that evening and silently watched TV together while Ethan slept on my lap. At 10 p.m., I decided to call it a night and went to bed.

Chapter 25

The Call

ETHAN WOKE AT ELEVEN CRYING TO NURSE, AS I was falling asleep. I pulled him into bed with me and lifted up my nightgown. Just as he began, my phone rang next to my bed. I froze. I knew this was it. I looked at the caller ID and saw the number from the hospital.

"Hello?" I whispered as I picked up, scared for what I was about to hear. I stroked Ethan's hair with my sweaty hands, as I waited for the news.

"Is this Allison?"

"Yes! Yes, it is," I said.

"I have good news for you, Allison. Listen carefully. We got a call for a heart, and your doctors think it is a perfect match for you. Now, the doctors went to go see the heart to look at it in person. They took a helicopter to Texas, since that is where the heart is right now. If it looks as good in person as they think, you will be getting your transplant soon!"

My hands started to shake. "Um, okay. So what do I do now? Should I pack a bag?"

"Don't worry about rushing too much. They are still in Texas. Why don't you pack a small bag for yourself and head over. Go to the ER and check in with the front desk. They will call for me."

I hung up the phone after we said our goodbyes. I did not want to get my hopes up. I had heard horror stories about people getting "the call," getting prepped for surgery, and the doctors realizing one small thing did not match up, then the surgery would be cancelled.

I walked into the living room holding Ethan in my shaking arms as he continued to nurse. "Dad?" I called out. He came out of the guest room, sleepy-eyed.

"They just called!" I said. Dad started to tear up. I had not seen him cry for as long as I could remember. I felt strangely calm. "It's okay, Dad. We have been waiting for this. It's going to be fine."

"Okay, okay, what do we do now?" he stammered, walking around in circles.

"Why don't I take a cab?" I could tell by how he was shaking that driving me and Ethan may not be the best idea. "Stay here with Ethan. I have some pumped bottles for him in the fridge. If you are freaking out, call the nurses on call so they can help you," I said, patting him on his back as I finished feeding Ethan.

We called for the cab, and I sat on the couch with Ethan in my arms, singing softly to him. I called Andrew to let him know I got my call.

"I love you so much. I can't wait to see you. You are going to do great, hon," he said, his voice shaking with emotion. If I got the team's approval to go ahead with surgery, he would book his flight to come down with my mom.

The cab arrived, and I held Ethan's face to mine and inhaled his sweet baby smell. "I love you, sweet boy. I'm doing this all for you." I was humming our song You Are My Sunshine, as I gathered my Ipad, a book, phone, my toothbrush, and pajamas in my backpack. I handed Ethan over to Dad, who was crying and shaking.

"Dad, call the nurses now to help you, okay? I'll see you soon. I'll call you as soon as I have any information." He hugged me and walked me down the hallway to the cab.

"Where to?" the driver said.

"Tampa General. I'm getting a heart transplant."

"A what?" he said. I giggled. "Well, I have never given anyone a ride for a transplant. Don't worry, I'll take good care of you and drive safely!"

I smiled in the backseat. "Thanks," I said. I let my hand glide over the sticky backseat as I looked out the window. For once, I didn't distract myself from the moment: no iphone, no music, no books. I was getting my heart.

Fifteen minutes later, we pulled up to the emergency room. I expected a team to be waiting for my arrival, whisking me into surgery as I had seen on television and in the movies. There was one woman sitting at a desk at the ER. She was fiddling on a cell phone. It was 12:30 a.m. I cleared my throat to get her attention. I was excited yet terrified, and eager to get prepped for the surgery.

"Um, excuse me?" She looked up. "I just got a call for a heart transplant?" I asked, as if it were a question. I waited for her excited response.

She sighed and handed me a clipboard. "Have a seat and fill this out. Someone will be with you shortly." Her eyes shifted back to her phone, and I chuckled to myself as I walked away, thinking, "I'm no big deal here in the ER."

I sat and waited. No one came for me. I called Dad to check on Ethan, and he said he had fallen back asleep. I breathed a sigh of relief, and then looked for the number to call the nurse who had called me earlier. "Hello? This is Ali Barton. I am in the waiting room at the ER."

"Oh, hi, Ali! That was quick. I'll come get you with a wheelchair," she said.

"I can walk, that's okay," I said, not quite ready to completely surrender yet. She had already hung up.

Minutes later, the wheelchair arrived. I was told the wheelchair transport was the protocol "just in case."

Chapter 26

Surgery

THE COORDINATOR WAS WHEELING ME AROUND the back hallways, and I felt frantic. It felt like she was taking forever. She even admitted at one point that she had gotten lost in the halls of the hospital.

"Did they say anything about the heart coming back yet from Texas?" I asked her as she rolled me into a small curtained room with a stretcher in it.

"The doctors are still there, Ali. My guess is they won't get back until early morning. Change into this gown and remove all your jewelry. We can put everything in security. You can keep your phone to update your family. We can give you something to relax if you think that will help you sleep. You need to rest up. Tomorrow will be a big day!"

"So we are not even sure the heart is good yet?" I screeched. "Ali, try to take some deep breaths. They wouldn't have gone to see the heart if they didn't think it was a great match. Try to stay positive."

As I changed out of my clothes, I started to panic. I sat down on the stretcher and called Andrew. "Hon, I don't think this is even happening until tomorrow.

There is no way I can wait all night! I am too anxious. I'm not going to be able to sleep at all!" I noticed my rumbling stomach. "And I am already hungry and have to fast before the surgery!"

Andrew laughed. "Priorities, huh? You'll be okay. Just keep us posted if you hear any updates. I'll book the flight as soon as you get the go-ahead."

A nurse came in to talk about the next steps. "This is looking good, Ali. So far, no news is good news. Now, how are you feeling?"

"I am so anxious! I don't think I'll be able to rest at all."

"Well, let's get your vitals and try to give you something that can help you relax and maybe rest a little bit." She started to take my blood pressure and her eyes widened.

"What's wrong?" I asked.

"Ali, I can't give you something to relax you. Your blood pressure is 70/50, and I think it is too risky to give you anything."

I sighed. I knew this meant no rest for me. I turned on the small television, and waited. I have no idea what was on TV, I just gave the screen a blank stare. The nurse took more information and then left the room again. I tried to rest but was unable to.

People ask me now if I was afraid of dying or not making it during the surgery. I was not. I just wanted to get it over with, and I had no doubt in my mind that I would be fine. They told me recovery could be difficult, and that the average hospital stay after transplant could be as little as a week, but was usually between ten to fourteen days. I knew I would be there for a week. I was young, strong, and otherwise healthy. I just wanted to get back to Ethan.

Hours later, a different nurse entered the room. "This looks like it is a go, Ali! Everything looks good. The doctors are on their way."

I texted the whole family with the news and then called Andrew. He booked a flight for himself and my mom. They would be there in a few hours.

"Do you know anything about the heart?" Andrew asked. I filled him in on what I had been told. The heart belonged to a young woman in Texas. It was not a high risk heart (meaning there was no drug overdose, Hepatitis C, or prostitution). Days later I found out that Andrew was watching the news on the flight down and saw the story about my donor's death. Everything matched up—she had been killed in a tragic accident involving other family members. I wasn't supposed to hear the details. I felt such an internal sense of shame about the waiting process. I had waited for months months, beginning in Boston, and this poor woman had died, allowing me to stay alive.

The rest of the morning was a blur. Several nurses prepared my body for the surgery. I remember lying on the table, looking up at the lights. The room was frigid, and I joked with them about how cold my breasts were exposed to the open air. I lay flat on the table, feeling blinded by the lights; I felt like I was on a movie set. Dozens of people walked around me, talking amongst themselves, and getting prepared. They painted my chest with a sterile solution, put an oxygen mask on my face, and a surgery cap over my head. I was anxious about not having weaned Ethan properly and wondered how he was doing with my dad at home.

I asked my nurse to have a breast pump ready for me in recovery. She laughed and said, "I think you are going to be a little bit out of it in recovery." And then I was asleep.

I woke up in the ICU surrounded by tubes and wires. Machines were beeping all around me and dozens of wires and tubes hung near my body. There was an IV line in my neck. As I tried to turn my head I felt a pull on my neck where my hair had been taped down with the central line. I felt thirsty, tired, and confused. Was the new heart in me? Was I alive? I tipped my chin down and saw white gauze on my chest, and realized the enormity of what had happened. I saw a glass wall in front of me, and looked to see Andrew pacing in front of my room. I could not speak, since there was a tube in my throat. I tried to lift up my hand to get his attention. I lifted it about three inches and gave a meek wave.

He looked up and locked eyes with me. "She's waving! Wow!" I heard him say to a nurse. "That's unbelievable!"

I tried to say hi. *I love you*, I thought. *Thanks for sticking with me, I know I've been a real pain in the butt.* Then I fell back asleep. All I wanted was something to drink.

I woke up again hours later, eager to get out of the ICU. My sister had arrived in town. Andrew was by my bedside, holding my hand. He had on a gown, mask, gloves and a hair cap. Anyone who visited me needed to cover up to avoid germ exposure. My immune system was so suppressed that contact with someone having a cold or dirty hands could turn into something deadly.

"I'm so thirsty," I said.

"Hon, they won't let you have anything to drink or eat because your stomach is full of air bubbles," Andrew said. "They have a tube in your nose to get some of the air out. They gave you Colace to help you go to the bathroom, since you haven't gone yet."

I shifted uncomfortably in the bed. "I want to get out of here. I can't move, I'm getting claustrophobic!" I said, getting more agitated. My heart started to beat fast, and it scared me into thinking something was wrong with this new one. It felt like it was pounding out of my sternum. "Where's Ethan?" I asked in a panic. "Who is he with? I want to see him!"

Andrew rubbed my shoulder. "Calm down, hon. Ethan is with your sister and dad. He's doing great. He's fine. You just need to get your rest and go poop so you can get out of here and onto a floor."

I started sobbing. "I miss him so much! I'm so thirsty!" Andrew walked into the hallway.

"Nurse?" I heard him ask. "She's really thirsty. Can she have a sip of water, or anything at all?" I heard the nurse murmuring to him, and Andrew walked back into the room holding a small cup with about two tablespoons of ice chips.

"Is that a joke?" I said, crying. "I need a cup of water! I'm so thirsty!" Andrew tried to calm me down, but I became hysterical. The transplant psychologist later explained to me that I had developed something called ICU psychosis, common in transplant patients. After the surgery is complete, a transplant patient is given a very high dose of steroids, which in and of itself can induce psychosis. Add that to being completely immobile in the ICU for days, unable to go the bathroom or do anything myself. It was the perfect combination for an emotional meltdown.

At the time, I did not know I had ICU psychosis. I was quick to spin out of control with my emotions, and my family could not understand what was happening to me.

Chapter 27

The ICU

I DON'T REMEMBER MUCH FROM MY WEEK IN THE ICU. As part of the psychosis, I remember yelling and fighting with nurses about being denied water. Certain nurses were younger and not as strict, and I would manipulate them to give me more ice chips than they should. I made sure my sister came with a bottle of my favorite flavor of kombucha when she came to visit me, just in case the doctors changed their minds and let me drink.

All I could think about was Ethan and kombucha. I face timed with Ethan every day and sobbed every time I saw him. I still had the air bubbles in my stomach, and I was not leaving the ICU until I had a bowel movement.

On the third day in the ICU, the nurses wanted me to get out of the bed. The physical therapist arrived just as I was begging Emily to sneak me some ice chips. "Hi Ali! I'm a PT here. How do you feel about getting out of bed and moving around a little bit?" I jumped.

"Really? I would love it!" I had high hopes for wandering the hallways and perhaps finding the ice machine without anyone noticing.

Emily held my hand. "You look so good, Ali. Your lips aren't purple anymore! Those last few months they were always purple. And your skin tone looks so good! You ready to do some laps?" I nodded, nervous to see how much strength I had lost. When they weighed me in the morning, I was 105 pounds, lighter than I had ever been. I knew my muscles had wasted away in those few months, and I felt weak and lightheaded from not eating anything. Emily grabbed one arm, and the therapist took my other arm. She attached a rope around my belly.

"You're going to walk me on a leash?" I joked.

"Nope! You're going to walk me. I'll stay a few feet behind just to be safe. The first rule of leaving your room is to get your mask, gloves, and gown on. The hospitals are the best place to pick up some kind of infection, and we want to prevent that."

The therapist had me practice how to sit up in the bed by rolling to my side and using my hand to push up. This was to prevent me from rising by using any muscles in my core or chest. Once I had successfully done this, she had me dangle my legs off the edge of the bed, and finally step down. It felt good to finally move my legs.

"Let's go," I said. "I want to walk!" Emily helped me with my protective clothing, and then got out her camera. She snapped pictures of me as I walked slow and cautious out of the room.

After the surgery, I had started a daily regimen of several anti-rejection medications that I would take for the rest of my life. I will always have a suppressed immune system, which will put me at risk to catch a virus or illness from someone else. The doctors also told me that it would make me more likely to have cancer in the future. I needed to be especially careful with sunscreen and with getting routine physicals and exams.

I did one loop around the ICU, going faster as I built confidence with each step I took. The nurses, the PT, and my sister cheered me on.

"Do you want to do one more?" the PT asked me. I kept my eyes open for the ice machine, but I was being watched so closely that I doubted I would be able to sneak any.

"Yes!" I said, elated to be doing so well this early on.

Emily laughed. "Of course she does. She's Ali!"

Two days later, I finally had a bowel movement. They were ready to move me to a recovery floor. Dr. Mackie and Tammi visited and were happy to hear how well I was doing. I begged them to let me drink the kombucha my sister had brought me.

"Ali . . ." Emily warned me, frustrated with my obsession with getting something to drink.

"Please!" I begged. "I will drink it slowly and only have half!"

Dr. Mackie agreed to let me drink half the bottle, just as Tammi rolled in a breast pump for me, borrowed from the labor and delivery floor. It had been several days since I last nursed Ethan. I was not as engorged as I thought I would be, most likely due to the diuretics I was being given at the time.

"I'm going to head out, Ali. Andrew is on his way. Glad you're doing so well! Love you!" My sister kissed me on the cheek. I was eager for her to leave. I wanted my drink, and I knew Emily would be monitoring how much I drank if she stayed.

I started to pump when everyone left the room. I had to dispose of the breast milk, since the medications I was taking could harm Ethan. I opened up the bottle of the kombucha. I smelled it and smiled. This was the first actual liquid to pass through my lips in almost a week. I took a small sip and knew I would be drinking the entire bottle.

My phone rang. Emily. I ignored it, ready to chug the entire thing. As I was finishing pumping, I felt a strange queasiness overtake me. The kombucha sloshed around in my stomach. It was going to all come back up. If I admitted what I had done, I would get a big "I told you so" from everyone. I looked into the pitchers I was pumping into. Since I had forgotten my pump bottles, I was using a large water pitcher for each breast. I vomited into the one I was holding in my right hand. Minutes later, the nurse stepped back in.

"All done with pumping?" she asked. I nodded.

"You can just dump these," I said, handing her the pitchers. I prayed that she would not look inside and see purple vomit mixed with the breast milk. The room was dim, and she was looking at my monitor as she dumped both pitchers directly into the medical waste bin. I sighed in relief.

Andrew walked into the room and kissed me hello. A few minutes later, I checked my phone to see that Emily had left me a message. It was: "Ali, don't you dare drink that whole bottle. Listen to your doctor. I know you too well." I laughed as I listened.

"Who was that?" Andrew asked, tilting his head.

"Just Emily, leaving me a silly message."

The next day, the seventh day with no food, the nurses said I would be able to go to a recovery floor if I could hold down some food. Andrew sat by my side as I requested a peach Greek yogurt and an orange. He peeled my orange for me, since my hands had a tremor from the medications.

I did not have much of an appetite, but said, "Oh, my God. This tastes amazing!" The orange and the yogurt went down with no problem, and the nurses began the paperwork to move me to a regular cardiovascular recovery floor.

Later that evening, I developed a ravenous appetite. The nurses assured me I could order dinner once I got to my room. I was still in my ICU psychotic stage, although unaware of it. When we settled into my new room and the nurse told me the kitchen was closed for the night, I almost lost my mind.

"You've waited this long, hon. You can just order something tomorrow," Andrew said.

I got angry. I was angry that I had to be in the ICU for so long, and angry that I was at Tampa General in the first place. I missed Ethan and I missed my life, and no one else could possibly understand how I felt.

"I have a protein bar in my backpack!" I suddenly remembered. "Yes!" I got so excited to unwrap the wrapper and eat, until Andrew interrupted my excitement.

"Ali, you should be gentle on your stomach right now after all that kept you stuck in the ICU. Those things can be really hard to digest. I think that's a really bad idea."

I scowled at him. "I'm eating it. I'm starving. I really don't care what you think." I started to take a bite.

"Fine," Andrew said, turning his back to me. "You clearly don't care if this messes up your stomach. You were in the ICU so long. Why mess around now?"

A nurse walked into the room as I yelled at him, "Fuck you. You can go. You don't understand." I sat down on the couch, unwrapping the wrapper to the bar. Andrew's built up stress hit the threshold.

"Fine! I'll leave! You don't care that everyone is trying to help you! Screw this. I'm leaving," he said as he turned to walk away.

I started to cry. We were yelling at each other, the pent-up months of fear and stress beginning to unravel. My prednisone rage and my psychosis did not help the situation; I found myself wanting to physically attack Andrew. *How dare he?*

The nurse stepped in. "You guys, I'm going to call security unless you both calm down."

With that, Andrew left the room.

Chapter 29

Recovery

THE NEXT DAY, ANDREW CAME BACK, FOLLOWED by the staff psychologist. I was weepy that morning, desperate to see Ethan and waiting to see if I would get approval for a visit. Angela had arrived in town and was with Ethan that morning. I had already done my daily face time sobbing routine earlier. The pain in my sternum from the cracking open of my ribcage paled in comparison to the pain of missing Ethan. I demanded my Dilaudid and IV Benadryl every four hours. Not for my chest pain, but to be numb and practically unconscious because I could not be home with Ethan.

According to the psychologist, the medications were making me behave like I was insane. "There is a condition known as ICU psychosis. I think the high doses of the prednisone and all of the transplant-related stress has made Allison a little aggressive," she explained.

Andrew and I glanced at each and giggled. "A little?" he said. We all laughed.

"I know I am crazy right now, hon," I said. "You can't listen to anything I say or do. I am so medicated and I feel nuts. I feel totally manic, like I can't sit still."

The doctor nodded. "This is common, Allison. As soon as the prednisone dose starts to come down, you will feel more like yourself."

Andrew held my hand. "She's had a tough time leading up to this. She's really independent and has wanted to keep her life as normal as possible. She doesn't like to let people help her. That's been hard. We were scared she could die any minute, and she had Ethan alone in her care."

I began to cry. "I know I'm crazy. But I don't think anyone else can possibly understand how I feel unless they've been through it themselves. I just want to see my son. I can't think about anything else," I said. My stomach churned, and I paced around the room as we talked.

"I think the doctors have given the okay for Ethan to come tomorrow," the psychologist said.

"Really?" I asked.

Every morning, I checked in with my mommy groups after I talked to my family. I was in two groups on Facebook for mothers of babies born around the same time. Band of Mothers and Tulips were some of my best supports during pregnancy. Even though I had never met many of the women, they were always sending supportive messages and sweet care packages to me.

Four of my closest friends in Tulips were Lauren, Erica, Janell, and Zayleen. We had talked every day since we had all conceived in the summer of 2013. These girls were my rock leading up to the transplant. That evening, I sent them the requested pictures of my "badass" scar.

While writing the girls a message and sending them photos, a nurse's aide came into my room to take my vitals and my weight.

"126. Hmm," she said. That was up twenty-one pounds from a few days ago. My heart sank. In the past, a gain like this meant something was very wrong with the heart. She paged my doctor. I was in a panicked frenzy.

Dr. Mackie came a few minutes later. "Allison, it's okay. This is normal after any kind of huge surgery like this. There are going to be massive fluid shifts. We will give you a few more diuretics and you'll see. Your body will balance back out."

I had been diligently walking laps around the hallways, eager to test out my new heart's capacity. But now I was scared that the surgery had not worked, or that I had already developed the dreaded rejection that everyone worried about.

He saw the panic in my eyes and put his hand on my arm. "Listen, we are keeping a good eye on you. Everything looks great right now. Your first biopsy was perfect. Just keep doing what you're doing." I nodded my head. "Is it true that your friend is coming to visit from Boston?" he asked, trying to lift my mood.

"Yes! One of my best friends, Emily! Is that still okay?"

My mood changed rapidly from minute to minute. I could go from sobbing to elated in a moment, and the thought of Emily visiting made me overjoyed. Dr. Mackie told me to get some rest, and that Emily could come over in the afternoon. "What about Ethan? Can I see him tomorrow?" He smiled and nodded his head, and I wept with joy. I was counting down the minutes to hold my baby.

Emily took a cab straight to the airport after her flight arrived from Boston. I had ordered her dinner from the cafeteria for when she arrived. The medications killed my appetite, and my old favorite foods sounded disgusting. Vegetables, meats, fish, and anything remotely nutritious repelled me. I was essentially living off yogurt, gluten free cereal, apples, and nut butter. I felt like I had felt during my pregnancy, like I had morning sickness all day long.

Emily was one of my favorite people to have around when I was sick, since she could always make me laugh and lift me out of a sour mood. We had talked a few days earlier about whether she should come or not. I had assumed I would be out of the hospital at this point, but she insisted she really wanted to see me and would love to help Andrew so he could get some sleep at night.

I wrapped my arms around her when she ran into my room saying, "Hey, mama!" It was so wonderful to see her. I had last seen her the day I said goodbye at the coffee shop. It felt as if years had passed.

We spent the night chatting, telling stories, and laughing about the vomiting kombucha into milk story. When a nurse came in to administer my medications and Ambien, she told Emily it was time to go. Emily stayed two more days before the rest of my family arrived and took the overnight shift with Ethan to let Andrew sleep. She planned on coming back in three weeks; I promised I would be more fun when I was out of the hospital.

The day after she left, my entire family was in town together. Dan and Holly came with Jake, along with my sister Emily and her fiancé Kate. That afternoon, everyone came to visit, along with our nanny Angela and Ethan. I had never been so excited in my life to hug Ethan. I heard a group of people walking down the hallway, and then heard the sweet familiar cry of Ethan as they got closer to my room.

"Hi, mama!" Andrew cheered, pushing Ethan's stroller though the doorway.

"Hi!" I jumped up from my bed to greet them. I was hooked up to an IV of magnesium and could only stand at my bed. Everyone was still required to put on a gown and mask. Andrew walked over and placed Ethan in my arms. My heart swelled with delight.

"This is where you are supposed to be," I whispered to Ethan as he gazed up into my eyes.

He was wearing a light blue onesie with no pants or shoes. He looked bigger than I remembered. I tickled his toes and smelled his skin as I kissed his face. "All of this was for you." His little hand reached for my chin, as I began humming to him. He fell fast asleep in the crook of my arm.

"The best part of this whole surgery is this part right now," I said. "Oh, how I missed this."

I had not seen Dan, Holly or Kate yet; they were shocked by the difference in the color of my skin and lips. I was so grateful to have my family all in one place, and I was excited to meet Angela in person. She was twenty-four weeks pregnant, and I knew Ethan would be in good hands based on the discussions I had had with her references. She would help me care for Ethan during my recovery, and I knew we would become friends. My worry about hiring help had been that Ethan would forget about me and think Angela was his mom. I needed the help, given how many follow-up appointments I would have after discharge. And I had strict instructions to not lift Ethan.

Angela was warm, funny, and she handled Ethan with great care. She gave me a huge hug, and after a few minutes of chatting, I realized I had found a true gem. She was a perfect fit for our family.

When Ethan woke up in my arms, the family took turns taking walks with me around the halls. No one, including myself, could believe how fast I could move and how easy it felt compared to years of huffing and puffing.

When they left, I felt the queasiness and rumbling in my stomach again, but tried to ignore it to go on my evening hallway walk. The OCD fitness nut in me was trying to walk a minimum of seventy-five minutes per day. I knew the stronger that I got, the earlier I would be discharged. I waved to my nurses as they praised me for my speed walking. On my fourth lap, I felt a sharp pain in my stomach and a gurgle.

"Uh oh," I said, biting my lip. With all the different medications I had been on over the last few years, I knew what that gurgle meant. I needed to get to the bathroom, and I needed to move fast.

I rushed back to my room and made it to the bathroom, but the explosion was so sudden that I did not make it quite to the toilet, and made a huge mess.

A nurse came running in after me. "Knock, knock! Ali?" she said, knocking on my open door.

"Don't come in! I'm too embarrassed!" I said, crying at the toilet. This uncontrollable sensation was how I'd felt when I had developed the serious colon infection, C. Difficil, in 2010. It was a common bacterial infection easily contracted in hospital settings, and the immune suppressed are more susceptible. The bacteria attacks the lining of the intestines and in serious cases can cause death.

I told the nurse, "I think I have C. Diff again. Can you get me some towels and cleaning stuff so I can clean this?" She stood in the doorway.

"Ali, don't worry! We see this stuff all the time. I'll have someone clean this up for you." She helped me wash off. The drugged up silly child in me couldn't help but snap a photo of my disgusting masterpiece to send to my girlfriends. To this day, they will not let me live it down. We go into hysterics every time we talk about my Tampa poop story.

The infectious disease doctor came in the following day to let me know that I had indeed tested positive for C. Diff. "You'll need to start the antibiotic Vancomycin tonight. I'm going to put an infectious disease precaution sign on the door of your room." I looked down at my hands, humiliated once again. "And I know this is going to make you upset, Ali, but I would suggest not having your baby come visit you until you finish the antibiotics."

My face fell. The idea of seeing Ethan once a day was what kept me going.

The doctor saw my disappointment. "I know this is tough, Ali. But his little immune system just would not be able to handle it if he got C. Diff. It would be devastating."

I nodded, understanding the risk and feeling depressed on a deep level. I thanked the doctor and called Andrew immediately, since they were planning to stop by later that day.

"Why does everything have to be so fucking diffi-cult?" I asked, calling Andrew, furious with this new diagnosis. "As if the transplant weren't enough, now I have to deal with this!" I would not be discharged until I finished the antibiotics; that added fourteen days to my stay. I'd been there almost two weeks. It was disappointing not to be one of the lucky trans-plant patients to leave a week after the surgery.

Andrew tried to reassure me. "In the grand scheme of all this, an extra two weeks will be noth-ing. Don't worry, hon. Dan will be coming soon, and I will come tonight after Ethan goes to bed."

I said nothing, drew the sheets up to my chin, and shivered in bed. Without Ethan, I didn't care about anything. It just hurt too much to feel.

My brother Dan came after I took my dose of Prograf, Cellcept, and prednisone. They were the main anti-rejection medications I would take twice a day for the rest of my life. There were other sup-plements and medications, but the doctors had been specific about taking these three twice a day, twelve hours apart on the dot. If I did not, I could risk my body identifying my new heart as a for-eign invader. If that happened, my immune system could build up antibodies that could eventually cause damage to the heart or cause an acute and dangerous rejection.

Rejection came in four levels: zero (the ideal, meaning no white blood cell inflammation on the heart tissue), one (meaning mild rejection, not usually treated but monitored) and two and three (more severe, and requiring IV medications and high dosages of steroids). I needed to be meticulous about my medication to avoid rejection.

Dan sat by my side as I swallowed my pills. We decided to take a walk when I was finished. I don't remember many specifics about the visits I had with my family during these weeks, as the pain medications make everything foggy. I remember Dan trying to cheer me up and make jokes as we took a walk around the hallways. He was leaving that night, but reminded me that I would be home in Boston before I knew it.

I was sure the C. Diff would push back my return to Boston. It was July 20th; I knew they would not let me go home to Boston in three weeks as I had hoped. One of my best friends Alexis had gone into labor the same night I got the call for the heart and the next day given birth to a beautiful baby girl. I was desperate to get home and visit her, but the reality was making that unlikely.

After Dan left, I asked my nurse for my Ambien and Dilaudid. Taking the medications felt better than the alternative: obsessing about going home to be with Ethan and Andrew.

The days passed in a blur. I overused the pain medications and IV Benadryl until I had finished the antibiotics. I did not want to be conscious. I was depressed, feeling nauseous from the medications, and I desperately wanted to go home.

After finishing the antibiotic, I tested clear for C. Diff. Dr. Mackie agreed to let me have a visit outside in the hospital pavilion with Ethan. It was my first time being outside in over two weeks, and I was instructed to wear my mask, gown, and rubber gloves. I knew I looked weird. People avoided coming close to me as I made my way downstairs, but I did not care. For once, I could see my family, hold my baby, and get an iced tea without counting how many ounces it was and making sure I "made it last" to fit into my fluid limit for the day.

The next day was my final biopsy of the week. If everything looked good, the doctors said I could be discharged. We spent the afternoon outside, enjoying family time in the sun. Ethan looked older and bigger to me.

"I want time to stop while I am gone! He's getting too big," I said.

"I bet you'll get out of here after the biopsy tomorrow," Andrew said, his blue eyes tired but smiling. I grinned. I felt great. I was feeling energetic and less swollen. All the post surgery fluid retention had come off, and for the first time in many years, I physically felt like myself.

I had my biopsy the following day then enjoyed another outdoors family visit to distract me from waiting for the results. I was nervous.

"This is make it or break it," I said to Andrew while I fed Ethan a bottle of milk. I wiped the drops of condensation from the cold glass bottle as Andrew rubbed my back.

"It will be a zero, hon. Look how great you're doing!"

Angela was sitting on the bench nearby. She looked at her watch. She had a doctor's appointment that afternoon.

"You guys should get going so Angela can get back on time." I smothered Ethan's face with kisses as he giggled his adorably raspy signature laugh. I gave a kiss to Andrew, hugged Angela, and left to go back upstairs. I would have given anything to leave with them.

Once I got to the room, I buzzed my nurse for pain medications. I just wanted to sleep until I could go home and be with my family.

The next morning, Dr. Mackie came in with Tammi and a group of doctors. Based on their facial expressions, I knew it was not good news.

"Hi, Ali. We got your biopsy results back, and it looks like you are going to be here a little longer."

I felt my eyes well up with tears. "What's wrong?" I asked.

"It looks like you have some 2R rejection going on. This is very common early on for people, particularly young people who are very healthy. Your body is smart and wants to fight off the new heart since it is foreign to your body. With you already in the hospital, we're going to treat this aggressively. There is an infusion called Thymoglubulin we'll give you for three days. The hope is that it will clear up the rejection and then we will let you go home."

"Is that different from the infusion I've already been getting?" I asked.

Once a week for ten weeks, I was to go to the cancer center to get a four-hour infusion, which would protect me from Cytomegalovirus (CMV). My donor was a carrier of CMV, and I was not. This is a potentially life threatening virus for immune suppressed patients. It was imperative I get these infusions to protect me and take a medication for six months called Valcyte. People who are immune suppressed can contract CMV, and it can have life threatening complications involving the eyes, lungs, liver, stomach, intestines, brain, and spleen. The infusions were imperative but exhausting.

"This is different, Ali. This is going to try and reverse the rejection. You will be hooked up to the IV for about eight hours each day. We will give it to you slowly and then adjust, since you seem to be reactive to these medications. We'll give you Ativan and Benadryl beforehand to hopefully ward off these reactions."

I nodded. I had been getting severe rigors with my infusions, where I would have violent shaking when the infusion started, like I was having a seizure.

"Can we get it started today? I want to be back home with Andrew for our wedding anniversary."

Our two-year anniversary was in a few days, July 28th. I was looking forward to celebrating out of the hospital.

"Ali, I think you are going to be here for at least another week. We really need to keep an eye on you." Tammi and Dr. Mackie glanced at each other. I braced myself for the next part of the conversation. "Ali, you won't be going back to Boston in a month like we had originally said. With the C. Diff and now this 2R rejection, we need you to recover a little longer in Tampa."

My stomach dropped, although I was expecting this decision. "Okay," I said, my voice shaking. I was devastated. I really liked my team and didn't want to annoy them, or make them think I wasn't grateful. What I really wanted was to hit someone and scream at the top of my lungs.

"If that is what you think I need to do, I obviously want to be safe."

My nurse gave me a look from the corner, where she stood at her laptop with my morning medications. I nodded, indicating that I wanted my Dilaudid. I suspected the nurses were aware that I no longer needed the high dose narcotics for sternal pain, but the prescriptions were still approved in the system. I didn't know how else to cope with my longing to be home. The days were long and boring, and I spent a significant amount of time obsessing about discharge.

The doctors finished explaining the infusion process to me. They felt confident it would reverse the 2R. Within twenty minutes, the infusion began, and I fell fast asleep with the help of the drugs.

Andrew and I celebrated our anniversary on the evening of my biopsy, after the three-day infusion. I eagerly awaited the results, since I would be discharged if they came back as a zero rejection.

Andrew surprised me with two dozen roses that evening. He was instructed to wear a gown, mask, and gloves. The flowers could not be near me because of potential bacteria. My immune system was even lower than it was in days prior.

"Well, this isn't exactly what I would dream about doing on my anniversary, but I'll take it!" I said, blowing Andrew a kiss. "I'm sorry I have put you through all of this, hon. I'll bet you never thought two years ago that you would be getting yourself into this kind of a mess. To say it has been stressful is an understatement."

He came and sat next to me on the bed. "In two years of marriage, we've made it through more than most couples will deal with in a lifetime. If we can make it through this, we can make it through anything."

I looked down at my scar, which was healing nicely. "I love you so much," I said.

"I love you too, hon. I bet this biopsy will be clear and you'll be coming home in the next few days."

Chapter 30

Discharge

THE NEXT DAY, TAMMI AND ANOTHER NURSE coordinator Lisa came in to tell me the biopsy was clear. "Looks like we can get the discharge paperwork started!"

"Really? Like I can go home today?" I asked, bouncing up and down in my bed. Lisa and Tammi nodded. I slid my breakfast tray over to the wall, and my yogurt and napkins splattered onto the floor. I could not contain my excitement.

"We are going to have Chrissy come by today with some pill boxes to go over all the medication instructions again today," Tammi said. I looked forward to a visit with Chrissy the pharmacist, a sweet and bubbly blonde woman who put great effort into ensuring that the medication brands I used would be gluten free.

With patience, she took hours explaining to me how to take the medications, and which foods and herbs I would need to avoid because of drug interactions.

"Okay." I nodded.

"Lisa is going to come by later when Andrew gets here so she can give you guys a little mini-guide to life after transplant. Things like how to avoid germs, when you need to come into the clinic, how to look for signs of rejection, and how to be careful eating out in restaurants."

I smiled. I was going home! The information was not overwhelming, though I couldn't help but think about how my life was going to be harder. I had done extensive research and participated in transplant forums, so I knew what life might look like after a transplant.

Our meeting later with Lisa confirmed what I already knew. I would need to be careful about germs; in crowded places I needed to wear a mask. I would need to carry hand sanitizer and Lysol wipes with me and wash my hands multiple times a day. I would take my medications morning, afternoon, and night for the rest of my life. Certain medications were to be taken separate from others to enhance the absorption. I was to take my temperature, heart rate and blood pressure twice a day and call the clinic if there were any changes. I was to weigh myself every morning, a habit I had deleted out of my life many years before I had gotten pregnant. The scale had way too much of an impact on my mood and was detrimental to my mental health. I did not plan on following up with the scale rule. Since I was very aware of when I was holding on to fluids, I'd weigh myself only in that case. If I was sick and vomiting, I was supposed to call the clinic. If I felt "off", I would call the clinic.

I was expecting the first year to be full of panic and anxiety, exacerbated by the fact that I would also be on high doses of prednisone which impacted my ability to sleep and function in a normal way. I would take Ambien to help me sleep at night. I was not allowed to drive for two months, since the impact of the airbag on my sternum could be problematic.

I would eat a lifetime diet of a pregnant woman: no raw fish, no unpasteurized cheeses, no buffets or salad bars, no raw foods in restaurants for a few months, no rare meats, no street foods or samples. The list felt like it went on and on, which was fine at that point since I had no appetite for any foods on that list. I was to make sure all fruits and vegetables were thoroughly washed, since there was a risk of E. coli and other bacteria. Any type of food poisoning or illness could send me straight to the hospital.

There were many rules that I wrote down as the nurses talked us. I noticed Andrew looking pan-icked. I put my hand on his leg, thinking, *Calm down, Andrew. We'll be fine.*

I was required to continue on my low sodium, healthy diet. I could return to the gym only during noncrowded hours, and I should sanitize everything I touched. I could not lift weights or do yoga for a few months until my sternum healed. I was eager to get back into fitness, so the thought of being back in the gym excited me. Despite the restrictions in my life, I was eager to walk around and not worry about my legs swelling or my lips turning purple.

Lisa explained the biopsy schedule. The doctor had a difficult time doing catheterizations through my neck, since there was excessive swelling post-surgery. Each week when I had a biopsy, I would be sedated, and the doctor would enter through my groin to enter my heart with a small catheter. Once the catheter was inserted, he would collect four to five samples of heart tissue to see if there were white blood cells present, which would indicate rejection. I preferred to go under sedation, as the procedure was extremely uncomfortable. For eight weeks, I would have one biopsy every week. Then I would have a biopsy every other week, four times. After that, they would be once a month, then every other month, then once every six months.

"If everything continues to go well, we hope you will be able to go home in October," Lisa said.

I was discharged from TGH on July 29th. I had been in the hospital nineteen days since the transplant. I had waited in Tampa for the heart for nineteen days. In thirty-eight days, my life had flipped upside down.

"I think it will go well. It has to be good luck that I waited nineteen days and was out in nineteen days," I said. Lisa and Andrew laughed.

"We hope so, Ali. Don't book the flights just yet, because we want to make sure you are in the clear for a while before we put you on a plane." Lisa had read my mind, as I planned on going on the Jet Blue website to book my flight for October 10, exactly three months to the day after my surgery. It felt like a lifetime away.

Later that evening, Andrew carried my belongings to the car. I made sure to thank and say goodbye to all my nurses. We had ordered a fruit and chocolate basket for them to enjoy, and I hugged my favorite nurses on my way out.

"Thanks for putting up with me all these weeks!" I said, half joking but mostly serious. I knew that prednisone made me crazy, the anti-rejection medications gave me stomachaches and migraines, and I was not in the best of moods during my recovery. The nurses had been amazing, taking great care to keep me comfortable and happy.

I insisted on walking down alone to meet Andrew at the car. I would not be rolled down in a wheelchair. I felt strongly about this. I promised myself when I had this surgery I would walk out on my own two legs, which is exactly what I did.

I was terrified.

Chapter 31

Home (in Tampa)

I CLIMBED INTO THE BACKSEAT OF THE CAR. Andrew turned around to look at me. From his seat, he grabbed my knee in excitement. It was a beautiful day. I looked at a palm tree as I inhaled the fresh air. I smiled at Andrew.

"This is awesome, hon! You're coming home!" he said.

I leaned back into my seat and relaxed. It was the first time in weeks that I did not have multiple monitors hooked up to my body and IV lines pumping medications into my arms. I felt elated but also naked and scared.

What would I do if something went wrong, with none of my nurses there? I was going home to take care of my baby, but who was going to take care of me? Tammi and Dr. Mackie had assured me I was ready to be at home. I physically felt excellent, with the exception of severe tremors from my Prograf and stomach upset and loss of appetite from the Cellcept. I had an excess of energy, partially due to being manic from the prednisone. I was tearing at the bits to get home to hold Ethan.

When we walked through the front door, Angela was on the floor playing with Ethan. "Welcome home!" she cheered with enthusiasm.

"Thanks!" I said. I had a moment of jealousy that she had spent every day with Ethan over the few weeks I was gone. I feared he would be more bonded to her than me. Looking at him made my eyes well up. His scrawny little legs kicked at his play piano gym mat. I couldn't wait to kiss him. I walked over to the living room and bent down to pick him up. I saw Angela shoot Andrew a nervous glance.

From the doorway, he said, "Hon, why don't you sit down and let Angela bring him to you? You're not supposed to be picking him up." I furrowed my forehead in annoyance.

Angela picked Ethan up and placed him in my arms as I sat down. "Here's mama!" she said. My heart melted. I was home.

Ethan tried to grab the gauze on my sternum; I redirected his hand into mine. "Mama's home! I missed you so much, my sweet boy." I started to cry. He had grown bigger over the three weeks I'd been away. I was heartbroken when he grabbed for my shirt to nurse and I had to refuse. The medications were too toxic and would pass through my breast milk. Andrew went to warm up a bottle.

"Do you need me to stay a little longer?" Angela asked. "That's okay, I think we're good," Andrew said. I could hear the familiar begging from our dog

Maddie in the kitchen. Ethan squealed when he heard her. I missed these little things. I was overjoyed to be out of the hospital and home.

Four days later, I had to say goodbye to Andrew. He had taken one month off work post-surgery, thanks to the Family Medical Leave Act (FMLA). I was devastated to see him go. The days leading up to his departure were spent on long walks with Ethan, lounging around by the pool, and ice cream dates. I wasn't ready to see him leave, though he would be back in two weeks. My parents would return the following day.

His last night in Tampa did not go as I had hoped. In the late afternoon, I started to feel nauseated, and then it escalated into a migraine. I could not move from a fetal position on the floor of the bathroom. I was terrified this meant I was in rejection. I was afraid of rejection from the moment I woke up in the morning until I fell asleep at night. Each morning, I stepped on the scale with my heart racing, nervous to see that old familiar increase of several pounds overnight. I was instructed to continue the diuretics, and I panicked each time that number rose on the scale.

That morning, the number was up one pound, which could mean the difference of how much water I had the night before, or if I had gone to the bathroom. When the uncontrollable vomiting started, I had Andrew call the team. Given that I had a few migraines while in the hospital, the team warned me that this could be a nasty side effect of the Prograf. They told Andrew to pick up a prescription for a migraine medication at our local Walgreen's.

I felt terrible. I vomited all through the night, and when there was nothing left in me, I sat near the toilet shaking and dry heaving. The team told Andrew I would need to come in if the vomiting did not stop. Luckily, it stopped when the sun began to rise. The medication kicked in, and I began my day as usual.

This soon became a part of my routine; one to two times a week of debilitating migraines, which I was assured would get better as my body adjusted.

"Ali, I think it is a good idea to go get labs just to make sure all your medication levels are okay," Andrew said, as he was heating up a bottle for Ethan.

"This is not how I want to spend our last day," I said, changing Ethan into a onesie and a new diaper. He looked up at me and cooed, and I stuck my tongue out at him. He laughed in his adorable raspy giggle that was my favorite sound in the world. "We'll go to Hyde Park and walk around after, get some iced coffee. It will be fun!"

We had discovered a fun area near the hospital that Dr. Mackie had suggested. It was full of local stores, coffee shops, and a charming park with a fountain. Every other Sunday, the entire area would shut down for a huge farmers and craft market, which we made sure to visit.

Spending time together as a "normal" family felt exhilarating, minus stopping for labs at the hospital. Towards the end of the day, my mood began to sour knowing that I would say goodbye to Andrew. I would be alone with Ethan for the first time, with strict instructions not to lift him, which was impossible. Ethan was sleeping in my bed when I was alone, so I could comfort him without leaning down into a crib to lift him.

As for not lifting him, I was a terrible patient. My weight lifting restriction was ten pounds; Ethan was thirteen pounds at six months old. Tell any mother she can't pick up her baby, and she would do the same thing.

Andrew was panicking about leaving, given the migraine incident from the night before. I promised him I would call Angela if I needed help and that she would be coming first thing in the morning. Ethan was not sleeping well, consistently waking three times after midnight. I knew I was in for a long night.

I called Andrew the following morning. "I did it!" I said with pride. For the first time since Ethan was born, I felt like a competent, stable, and healthy mom.

"He woke up so many times in the middle of the night, but I don't even care! I did it," I said, as I bounced Ethan on my lap. He tried to pull on my sternum gauze, and I handed him a rattle. I tickled his belly as I heard Angela coming in the front door. I sighed. I loved Angela, but hated that I had to rely on someone to help me. I wanted to be fully independent, although I knew I had my limits. Despite being hyper and manic on the prednisone, I was also easily exhausted with a tendency to overdo it. I was unable to drive for two months and had to get to my follow up appointments. Angela was helpful and considerate about giving me my independence, and we came to grow close in the following weeks.

"Mom and dad will be here later today, so I will give you a call after they settle in. Love you, bubs. I miss you already," I said.

"Love you too. Please try to take it easy, hon. Let people help you."

Ha. Easier said than done.

Chapter 32

Back to Normal

LIFE WENT BACK TO AS NORMAL AS IT COULD BE in the following weeks. I went to the hospital every few days for my CMV infusion, a biopsy, a clinic visit, or labs. My parents came, followed by my friend Emily, then my sister. We had busy days full of long walks, coffee shops, ice cream, farmers' markets, pool time (not above the waist for me), and visits to the gym.

It was eerily similar to being on vacation, except I was desperate to go home, not to mention the frequent incidents of becoming violently ill from the medications. Because of the prednisone mania, I spent a lot of time overdoing it, moving around too much, and pacing the hallways back and forth for hours so Ethan would nap in his stroller.

The heat in Tampa was unbearable in August. We made our best effort to not spend time outside between the hours of 10 a.m. and 4 p.m. The hallways were shaded and cool. They allowed me to get my jittery energy out while Ethan was refusing any kind of nap in his crib.

I thought about the heart frequently. I couldn't believe how much energy I had at my first gym visit. I stepped on the elliptical machine and pedaled for forty-five minutes, which I hadn't done in years. Before the surgery, after twenty minutes my legs would start to swell, and I would be exhausted as if I had run a marathon.

Weeks after the surgery, I didn't recognize the woman I saw in the mirror at the gym. I had pink in my cheeks and my lips were not blue. I looked happy and healthy. I couldn't believe how lucky I was to get transplanted within weeks. Ethan would sit in his stroller by my side, or play with toys on a towel next to me in the empty gym, watching my every move. I would sing him songs and make funny faces, astonished that I could sing and exercise without gasping for air. I felt happy and free.

That is the tough thing about transplants. One part of me felt (and feels to this day) overwhelmed with gratitude for new heart; and the other part feels a desperate sadness that someone had to lose her life to save mine. I think about my donor every single day, and I talk to her often in my mind.

At times I feel livid that any of this happened to me. Why should a thirty- two-year-old need a new heart? After connecting with many other transplant patients in the last few years, I came to realize this is a common phenomenon.

I struggle with guilt for feeling angry at my situation. I have come to accept that I can feel grateful for my donor, yet angry that I lost so many years of my life to my heart condition. I am angry that I have always tried to take good care of myself and be healthy, while I still needed a new heart and I had a premature baby. I don't think I can ever let go of my anger about getting sick; I think accepting the anger is a very important part of the process.

Getting sick is hard for someone who is a control freak. Your body is doing something that feels wildly out of control, and nothing you say or do can change it. I continue to have resentment today. Prednisone caused me to gain about fifteen pounds, despite my best attempt to stay fit and watch my diet. It can be frustrating to feel like nothing I do works, and that my body is an uncontrollable thing.

It was traumatizing for me to be an observer as I got sicker. It would be a long process to heal my mind and recover from this trauma. It was helpful to have visits from my family and friends while I was in Tampa. Staying busy was imperative to keeping me from feeling sorry for myself.

Luckily, Ethan kept me on my toes during this adjustment time in Tampa. He was just starting solid foods; making batches of homemade purees to freeze was turning into a fun and distracting activity for myself. I had no appetite when they increased my dose of Cellcept. All food sounded disgusting to me. Most days, I would make a meal, and then feel nauseous when I sat down to eat it.

Not wanting to waste food in the freezer purchased prior to the transplant, I decided to make purees for Ethan. I first tried organic chicken blended with broth. I thought I was genius for creating this healthy meal, but neglected to think about how nauseated I would get when trying to feed it to Ethan. When I took one whiff of the chicken, I began to cough and dry heave. That meal choice was delegated to other people to feed to him. I would get sick just thinking about that particular blend.

We went to the local frozen yogurt store on most days, since yogurt was the only thing that sounded appetizing to me. I would spend about ten dollars on a cup of yogurt the size of my head, and that would be my main meal for the day.

The weeks passed slowly. I was desperate to get home to Boston. My family took turns coming down, and we had some great day trips to local beaches and restaurants. Many nights I would cry on the phone to Andrew about being homesick. At my next clinic visit, I decided to ask Dr. Mackie if he had any updated information on when I could go home.

"If there are no more episodes of rejection and if everything continues to go smoothly, we are willing to send you home at the three month mark," he responded. "But we will want you to have a follow up at Brigham and Women's as soon as you get home. We have to keep an eye on your Prograf and white blood cell levels." My Prograf levels had been fluctuating wildly. The doctors had given me a shot called Neupogen to raise my white blood cell counts.

Over the weekend, I developed hives all over my body. They determined it was an allergic reaction to the shot. There was no other way to raise my white blood cells.

"We are going to take you off the Valcyte, since that lowers your white blood cell counts to virtually nothing," Dr. Mackie explained. The Valcyte was another preventative medication to keep me from getting the CMV that my donor carried.

"The infusions should keep you from getting CMV, but you are going to have to be extremely careful about germs when you get home. Wear your mask, wash your hands a lot, and bring hand sanitizer everywhere you go. Getting CMV would set you back a lot. People feel pretty terrible when they get it. If you notice a stomach bug, fever, or generally feeling terrible, call your team. It's always a good idea to call your team if you have any concerns. You know you can always call us too. I hope you consider us your team, even though you are going back home to Boston. Though I think you and Andrew should move down here. I'm just saying . . ." Dr. Mackie said with a chuckle and a smile.

I laughed, knowing that this team felt like family to me and I would always be in touch with them.

I panicked for a moment after, thinking about the weird looks I would get in public with the mask. I supposed that would be better than full body hives.

"Hopefully, just coming off the Valcyte will allow your white blood cells to come back up," he continued, as I mentally calculated the date for the flight I would be booking.

Surgery had been July 10th. October 10th was the three-month mark. A few weeks away! The flight was booked in the car ride home from the hospital.

Chapter 33

Shipping up to Boston

ANDREW WAS FLYING DOWN THE FOLLOWING day to help us home. It was a Friday evening. I had packed up the entire car full of our belongings, ready for the transport truck taking my car home to Boston to come get the car. I had had an argument with the original transport company. A truck part was broken; without a replacement, they would not be able to take my car back to Boston for another week. In a panic, I had scrambled to find another company. They were charging me an arm and a leg, but I didn't even care.

After putting Ethan down for his bedtime, I got a call from the driver. "Ms. Barton? I can't get to you. There's a sign on West Shore Boulevard saying no trucks allowed. The trees are too low and my truck won't fit. I'm going to need you to come meet me. I'm about two miles down the road."

The car was filled from top to bottom, with no room to fit Ethan in his car seat. I started to cry. I was alone; Angela was out for the evening. "Can you hang tight for a few minutes? My son is asleep, and I am alone here."

He agreed to wait for ten minutes to see if I could find a solution. I had no clue what to do but decided to knock on my neighbor's door. Although I did not know them well, they were a nice military couple, and I was desperate.

The husband was in his pajamas. I explained what was going on and asked if they were willing to sit with Ethan as he slept. My plan was to jog the two miles home after dropping my car off. The husband insisted on following me and giving me a ride back. I breathed a sigh of relief and thanked them. They followed me into the apartment as I called the truck driver to let him know I was on my way.

When Andrew came the following day, I was a nervous wreck. I had been waiting weeks to go home. Now that it was time, I was not sure I was ready. Andrew tried to help me as I attempted to stuff our belongings into one suitcase. He realized that the best idea might be to give me some space, since I snapped at him every time he said anything.

I wanted to see my friends and family when I got home, yet I was terrified of germs and getting sick. I was in a clean little bubble in Tampa and not around small children who could be sick. I wanted Ethan to have a normal life full of play dates and fun activities, but I was also scared to land myself in the hospital by exposing myself to baby coughs and runny noses.

Prior to leaving Tampa, I had sent an email to friends and family explaining my suppressed immune system and extremely low white blood cell counts, and my need to be cautious. I begged people to not visit me if they had been sick, had been near a sick person, or thought they may be getting sick. Everyone agreed to be very respectful and cautious of this.

As I packed up my Tampa life into one big red suitcase, I realized I would miss it there. I loved the people, the area, and the activities. I had grown close with Angela and my transplant team, and I'd had a fun time recovering in Florida. The weather was finally nice, as October is one of the best months to be there. I was dreading winter in New England and wondered if it was actually a good idea to go home.

The next day, I sat in a wheelchair in the Jet Blue terminal, holding Ethan in my arms while he slept. People stared at my mask with nervous glances. When we arrived at our terminal, we realized that Andrew had not received his boarding pass and would need to run back to check-in to get it. In September and October, there had been an Ebola outbreak, and the airports were strict about who could fly. People glared at me as I sat alone in the chair, wishing Andrew would hurry. I joked around with Andrew that I should have a label on my mask saying, "It's not me, it's you." Luckily, the flight went seamlessly and Ethan slept for the entire time.

We made it. I was home. It was a warm fall day in Boston. Walking into my house for the first time in four months felt amazing. I was grateful to have made it home in one piece. Ethan squealed as Maddie jumped up to greet him.

"We're home!" I yelled to no one in particular. Andrew chuckled. He carried our bags into the house and I placed Ethan onto his play mat.

"Feel good?" Andrew asked, rubbing my back.

"It feels awesome! But I'm also really scared. I want to see so many people, but I am also afraid of getting sick. I just want a big bubble for me and Ethan."

"It will be okay, hon. Everyone knows how weak your immune system is now. They're smart enough to keep their distance if they are sick," he said as we watched Ethan fiddling with toys. Ethan giggled and looked up at us, and my eyes filled with joyful tears.

When we had left Boston, he could barely lift his head off the ground; now he was sitting independently and playing with his toys. I glanced over to see our brown glider chair in the corner. I had spent many hours in that chair breastfeeding Ethan. It was a painful reminder that I could no longer feed my baby in the way I wanted to.

Andrew read my mind and said, "I can move it upstairs later. Let's get some dinner."

The following few days were filled with visits from my family and my best friends. It was wonderful to see everyone I had missed while I was away but overwhelming at the same time. At times I felt like crawling under the covers and isolating myself from the world. Although I realized the medications altered my cognitive processing, it was hard to get around the mood swings that I felt with the prednisone.

I was scheduled to have a doctor's appointment three days after getting home to Boston. At that appointment, we discovered my medication levels were off and required some adjusting. This went on for the following year: my medications never stayed stable and were constantly adjusted. This later required a three-day hospitalization to take labs every few hours to evaluate my absorption issues. The doctors and lab visits were frequent in those first few months as my body adjusted.

When I went to the hospital, I visited my old floor on Shapiro to see my nurses from when I was pregnant. Going back to Brigham and Women's still triggers anger in me to this day. The traffic, the busyness, the long waits for appointments; an anger stirs up deep within me, and I want to cry every time I go. This requires deep breathing, sometimes taking anxiety medication. I love my nurses and the team, but I will always see it as the place where I was told to give up on Ethan. I thank God that I refused their medical advice.

When Ethan joins me at an appointment, I feel like holding him up to everyone and saying, "See what you wanted me to give up? Thank goodness I ignored you all!"

I spent most of the winter at home with Ethan, rarely going into public places out of fear. I got sick a few times and had health scares. Any scary symptom makes me believe I am in rejection. I will never experience heartburn in the same way I used to before my transplant. A transplant patient never takes chest pain lightly.

One night I had severe chest pain in January, 2015. Andrew called 911 in a panic, and the ambulance came to take me to Brigham. I had insisted it was heartburn, but a small part of me was terrified that something was wrong. While anything serious was ruled out at the hospital, I was still forced to spend the next two days there with the resulting migraine that left me vomiting dozens of times.

I had another hospitalization a few weeks later from catching the stomach flu from Ethan. The doctors had told me I needed to stay away from Ethan if he were to get sick, but as a stay at home mom it is impossible to not be puked or pooped on. When I got his flu, I could not keep my medications down and spent a few days on IVs in the hospital.

Chapter 34

Life

THE REJECTION. THERE HAVE BEEN MULTIPLE EPIsodes of mild rejection. Things would get better, and they would wean me off prednisone only to put me back on it at the next biopsy. The rejection was infuriating. Normally I felt great, with no typical symptoms of rejection like low blood pressure, fever, rapid weight gain, or feeling exhausted. It was always a surprise to me when the clinic would call with the bad news. Finally, I got used to it, and realized that mild rejection is common in young, healthy people. Since I have autoimmune disease, my body is also more apt to recognize something foreign in my body as an invader.

Overall, life has been amazing post-transplant. Minus the worst winter in Boston's history, it was great to be back home.

At the one-year mark, we had an Organ-niversary party with all our friends to celebrate. I felt so blessed to have such wonderful friends and family close by. Many of my friends also stayed home with their children. My days were filled with play dates, early intervention activities, music classes, and baby/mommy fitness groups. Mama Beasts was one of these.

Mama Beasts became one of our favorite activities. It was where I learned I could be athletic again. I surpassed my level of fitness from before I got sick. Ethan could run around like a maniac with the other children. It was a great way for us to meet friends who had similar interests. The women I have met in Mama Beasts have been remarkable, and the children have a blast together.

Andrew and I decided last year that we would love to have another child. My doctors are not enthusiastic about another pregnancy for me. The medications I take are known to cause birth defects in babies, and the chances are high that I would go into a significant rejection if we made any changes with the medications.

On a more personal note, I know the tragic story of the woman who died and gave me he heart. I feel like it would be disrespectful to her and her family if I were willing to risk harming the heart that she gave me. I would carry a tremendous amount of guilt knowing I did not do my best to take care of her precious gift.

We began to discuss the option of using a surrogate, and I began my research in the summer of 2015. A friend who was a surrogate recommended posting my story in a group for intended parents and surrogates that she was involved with. I shared my story, hoping to avoid the fees of using a surrogacy agency. I wanted to find someone on my own.

Jess reached out to me after I shared my story, and we hit it off. We made plans to talk on the telephone first. We chatted for an hour, having a lot in common. We made plans to meet in person, to meet at the zoo one afternoon with her three children and Ethan. Within ten minutes of being with her, I knew I wanted her as my surrogate. She tells me she felt the same connection and thus began our journey.

Since then, we had an intense two-day long screening at my fertility clinic, where Jess underwent several medical tests and psychiatric screenings. We had group social work sessions with Jess, her husband Jamie, Andrew, and myself. She was approved, and we could not be happier.

I was nervous to do IVF again, since I always had a poor yield. My doctor suspected it was because of the undiagnosed heart failure, with my body's organs struggling as a result. Sure enough, when I cycled in April 2016, we produced a high yield of embryos with normal chromosomes. We went through one cycle in July that failed, but the cycle in September was successful. We are officially pregnant with a little girl. Since we biopsied the embryos, the embryologist told us the gender at the transfer. Jess is due with our baby in May of 2017. I am blessed to have met such an amazing woman.

I have a lot of mixed feelings about not being able to carry my baby myself. Knowing I can't carry my baby makes me feel like weeping at times. It triggers a greater resentment for everything I have been through, and how this heart has ripped away my ability to do one of the most natural things a woman can do. I mourn this loss.

I missed having the pregnancy where I could be out in public, enjoying the attention pregnant women get, relaxing on my couch, getting foot rubs and taking baths. I spent my pregnancy in a hospital gown, stressing about when my heart was going to give out and if my baby would live.

I can be happy for my friends who conceived the "easy" way, but a small part of me hurts when I see someone else pregnant. I hate that I had to miss out on the experience of a normal pregnancy, and I can never get that back. I can't let myself get too deep into these emotions, as I know it is not beneficial to me. All I can do is thank my lucky stars that I met Jess when I did and how I did. It was meant to be. Jessica's family has become part of our family, and the gift she is willing to give us is magnificent. It takes a selfless and remarkable woman to offer her body to carry a baby. I have been lucky enough to embark on that journey with Jess. We are excited to give Ethan a sibling, and I know he is going to be an amazing older brother. Ethan asks for "baby sister" every time he sees another baby. I say, "We have to wait, honey," and he replies, "Jess is making her!" It warms my soul.

For me, it has to be about moving on and moving forward, without forgetting or denying my past. If I stop and let myself sit in the negativity and the memories, I go to a dark place. I think of my transplant as a part of me that I can't change, even though I wish I could take away the pain and anxiety I have caused loved ones over the last few years. The transplant and my pregnancy prove to me that I am strong, passionate, optimistic, and perseverant. When I make up my mind about something that is important to me, I know I can follow through and always trust this new heart of mine. I am always surrounded by love and support, and that is what keeps me going.

This transplant was a gift. Ethan's full name, Ethan Matthew, means "strong gift from God." After all we have been through, it holds true. I have been given many gifts from God: Ethan, Andrew, my family, my donor, finding Jess, our baby girl, and my new heart. I am completely blessed.

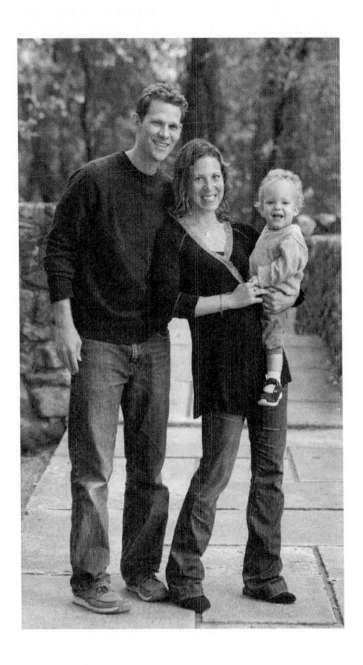

About the Author

ALI BARTON IS A LICENSED PSYCHOTHERAPIST and wellness coach with a private practice outside of Boston, Massachusetts. Currently, her most important job is a stay at home mom to her son Ethan, who was born months before Ali had her heart transplant in the summer of 2014. Ali has always been interested in health and fitness, especially after getting sick with multiple autoimmune diseases related to undiagnosed celiac disease in 2010—Hashimoto's thyroiditis, ulcerative colitis, and an undiagnosed heart condition. When Ali got pregnant with her doctor's approval in 2014, her autoimmune disease spiraled out of control, and her heart went into failure. Doctors recommended that she end her pregnancy at twenty-one weeks, and she refused to do so. Her son Ethan was born prematurely at thirty-one weeks, and is thriving today! She had her heart transplant at Tampa General Hospital when Ethan was six months old.

After her experience, Ali felt strongly motivated to write about her story, especially about trusting your gut and advocating for yourself in a medical setting. She blogs at www.aliweinbergbarton.com.

Acknowledgements

I NEVER WOULD BE HERE TODAY IF IT WERE NOT for the endless amount of love and prayers from my friends and family.

To my family: Mom and Dad, who came to visit every single day for months—I don't deserve you. I can't tell you how much that helped me get through. Emily and Dan—you are my rocks. I love you guys so much.

Holly, Kate, Jakey, Stelle, Zayde, Marilyn, Aunt Corinne, Uncle Jan, Ellen, Ray, Chris, Ange, Beth, Julia, Riley, Susie, Jimmy, Susan, Erica love you all!

My friends at Stil Yoga (Kevan and Betty) and Sarah Andres Gardner: When you created Rally for Ali when I was twenty-two weeks pregnant, I was honored and in shock at the same time. Your support through everything—from helping me cope with my infertility all the way to heart failure and heart transplant will always stay with me. Thank you for making so many things possible for me. Thank you for helping me stay calm and strong in moments of utter terror.

My friends who have supported me in my darkest moments, visiting me in the hospital and always standing by my side, I will never forget it. You pulled me through.

Emily, Tracy, Alexis, Tricia, Linda, Ilana, Michelle L, Michelle G, Dan, Mike, Lesley, Rachel, Dana, Lauren, Erica, and Janell. To my Tulips and Band of Mothers, thanks for always being there and supporting me. My Mama Beasts—you keep me strong and on my toes. Antoinette, thank you for bringing together this amazing group of moms and kids.

My transplant sisters and brothers—especially Elissa, John and Susan, Keilah, Heather D., Heather I., Grace, June and Al, Edwina, Ali, Andrea, Sherrette, Paula, Natalie, Tammy, and Darlene. Thank you for your endless support, answering my questions and worries twenty-four-hours a day in our survivor group. I couldn't get through it all without you.

Elissa and Natalie, you spoke with such eloquence before my transplant and made me feel completely comfortable and confident in my decision. I panicked before I talked with you both. Thank you for sharing your stories.

Jessica—thank you for coming into my life and helping us to bring another baby into this world. You are an amazing, wonderful woman. I am so lucky to have met you.

Angela, thank you for watching my baby in Tampa. I never worried when Ethan was in your care, and you made an isolated post transplant experience and a scary situation feel good for me.

Donate Life New England for allowing to me work with you and share my story to spread organ donation awareness.

To my medical team in Tampa, especially Dr. Ben Mackie, my heart surgeons, and Tammi Wicks—you are my heroes. And thank you to Lisa, Kim, and Chrissy, and to all of my nurses at TGH. Thank you for saving my life and for making me smile throughout the process.

To the doctors and nurses in the NICU, especially Felicia—thanks for saving my baby. You all are amazing.

To my medical team at Brigham and Women's, especially my wonderful nurses, and Dr. Lakdawala, Dr. Stuart, Dr. Givertz, Dr. Mehra, Dr. Nohria, Dr. Economy, Dr. Smith, Dr. Little, Erica, Kathy, and Debbie. Thank you for putting up with me and supporting me (even when I was being stubborn and crazy), and for keeping both me and Ethan safe when I was pregnant. To Chrissie, Marie, Sheri, Clare, Katherine, Morgan, Karen, Wylie, Amy, Jill, Jackie, Ashley, Claire, Alyson, Heather, Lauren, Debbie, Karen, Gretchen, Mary, Danielle, and Ally. Thanks for making me laugh when I wanted to crawl in bed, give up and cry.

To the moms who generously donated milk to Ethan--especially Amanda, Emily, Bridget, and

Kristina. You helped make Ethan healthy and strong when I could not do it myself anymore.

To WiDo Publishing—especially Allie Maldonado and my editor Karen Gowen-- thank you for taking a chance on me. I am honored and thrilled to work with you.

To Judy Gelman, for all of your help and advice. I never would have had the courage to get published if it were not for you.

Andrew—I love you. The man who stands by a woman's side throughout all of this is a hero in my book. Here's to the rest of our lives hopefully being a lot calmer. You are my best friend and I'm sorry that I made us both age twenty years in the last two years!

Ethan: my sweet, kind, delightful, smart boy. I did this all for you, and I would do it a million times over again. You are my world, and I could never be as happy as I am now without you. In my wildest dreams, I never could imagine what a joy you are. Thanks for being my best little bud.

My donor: Thank you for giving me a second chance at life. You are selfless and incredible for checking that box on your license, and you will always be part of me. I think about you every day. Thank you for the gift of my life.